Public Health Leaders Tell Their Stories

Lloyd F. Novick, MD, MPH
Carol Spain Woltring
Daniel M. Fox, PhD

D1566241

An Aspen Publication®
Aspen Publishers, Inc.
Gaithersburg, Maryland
A Copublication with the Milbank Memorial Fund
1997

Library of Congress Cataloging-in-Publication Data

Novick, Lloyd F.
Public health leaders tell their stories / Lloyd F. Novick, Carol
Spain Woltring, Daniel M. Fox.
p.   cm.
Includes bibliographical references and index.
ISBN 0-8342-0961-6
1. Public health administration—United States—Case studies.
2. Public health—Political aspects.   I. Woltring, Carol Spain.
II. Fox, Daniel M.   III. Title.
RA445.N68   1997
362.1'0973—dc21
97-15629
CIP

With the exception of Chapter 14, which is in the public domain, all of the chapters in this
publication are articles that have been reprinted from issues 3:1 and 3:4 of the *Journal of
Public Health Management and Practice* © 1997, Aspen Publishers, Inc.

Orders: (800) 638-8437
Customer Service: (800) 234-1660

About Aspen Publishers • For more than 35 years, Aspen has been a leading professional
publisher in a variety of disciplines. Aspen's vast information resources are available in
both print and electronic formats. We are committed to providing the highest quality information available in the most appropriate format for our customers. Visit Aspen's Internet
site for more information resources, directories, articles, and a searchable version of
Aspen's full catalog, including the most recent publications: **http://www.aspenpub.com**
Aspen Publishers, Inc. • The hallmark of quality in publishing
Member of the worldwide Wolters Kluwer group.

Editorial Resources: Sandra L. Lunsford
Library of Congress Catalog Card Number: 97-15629
ISBN: 0-8342-0961-6

Printed in the United States of America

1   2   3   4   5

Table of Contents

About the Contributors

Kaye W. Bender, MS, RN is Chief, Office of the State Health Officer, Mississippi State Department of Health.

Bobbie Berkowitz, PhD, RN, FAAN is Deputy Director of the Robert Wood Johnson Foundation "Turning Point" National Program Office at the University of Washington, School of Public Health and Community Medicine. She has also served as the Deputy Director of the Washington State Department of Health and the Chief of Nursing Services for the Seattle-King County Department of Health.

Jack Dillenberg, DDS, MPH is Director of the Arizona Department of Health Services and is the President of the Association of State and Territorial Health Officials (ASTHO) in 1996–1997.

Grace G. Eddison, MD is the Acting Chairperson for the Gateway Regional Interagency Delivery System (GRIDS). She has also served as the Commissioner of Health, Gateway District Health Department in Owingsville, Kentucky.

Daniel M. Fox, PhD is President of the Milbank Memorial Fund. His most recent book is *Power and Illness: The Failure and Future of American Health Policy* (Berkeley: University of California Press, 1995).

Kristine M. Gebbie, DrPH, RN is the Elizabeth Standish Gill Assistant Professor of Nursing and Director, Center for Health Policy and Health Services Research at Columbia University School of Nursing. She also serves as a Senior Consultant on Public Health Initiatives to the Office of Public Health and Science, U.S. Department of Health and Human Services. She was previously the first National AIDS Policy Coordinator, appointed by President Bill Clinton, Secretary of the Department of Health for the State of Washington, and the Public Health Administrator for the State of Oregon.

Fernando A. Guerra, MD is Director of Health, San Antonio Metropolitan Health District in San Antonio, Texas.

Douglas Hirano, MPH is a Special Assistant for Public Health Policy and Practice for the Arizona Department of Health Services.

Susan J. Klein is the Director, Division of HIV Prevention, AIDS Institute of the New York State Department of Health.

John C. Lewin, MD is Executive Vice-President and Chief Executive Officer of the California Medical Association. He has also served as Director of Health for the State of Hawaii, the Chief Executive Officer of Hawaii's largest hospital system, and President of the Association of State and Territorial Health Officials (ASTHO). He previously directed the Navajo Tribal Division of Health Services.

Charles Mahan, MD is Dean of the College of Public Health and Professor of Obstetrics and Gynecology at the University of South Florida. He has also served as State Health Officer in Florida and as President of the Association of State and Territorial Health Officials (ASTHO).

Thomas L. Milne is the Executive Director of the Southwest Washington Health District, Vancouver, Washington.

Lloyd F. Novick, MD, MPH is Commissioner of Health of Onondaga County and Professor, Department of Medicine, SUNY Health Science Center in Syracuse, New York. He has also served as First Deputy Commissioner for the New York State Department of Health, the Secretary of Human Services and Commissioner of Health for the State of Vermont, and Director of Health Services for the State of Arizona.

David R. Smith, MD is President of the Texas Tech University Health Sciences Center. He has also served as the Commissioner of the Texas Department of Health and Senior Vice-President of Parkland Memorial Hospital in Dallas.

Martin P. Wasserman, MD, JD is the Secretary of the Maryland Department of Health and Mental Hygiene. He has also served as the Health Officer for Prince George County and Montgomery County in Maryland, and as Director of Human Services for Arlington County, Virginia.

Paul J. Wiesner, MD is Director of the DeKalb County Board of Health in Decatur, Georgia.

Carol Spain Woltring is the Director of the Public Health Leadership Institute and the Center for Health Leadership in Berkeley, California. She has also served as Public Health Administrator for the Contra Costa County Health Department and as Deputy Director of the Health Officers Association of California.

Foreword

The Milbank Memorial Fund is an endowed national foundation that supports nonpartisan analysis, study, and research on significant issues in health policy. The Fund often makes available the results of its work in pamphlets and books, and it has published the *Milbank Quarterly,* a peer-reviewed journal of public health and health care policy, since 1923.

This book is the result of a collaboration between the Fund and the recently established *Journal of Public Health Management and Practice.* This journal is written and edited by and for persons who do the daily work of public health, especially in government at all levels but also in voluntary agencies and other private organizations.

The stories about public health leadership in this book are first-person accounts that were reviewed by other leaders. The stories are neither confessional nor sensational because each of the authors adheres to standards of confidentiality and caution that are prerequisites for professional careers in the public sector. Nevertheless, each story is vivid and informative. We appreciate the significant effort that each of the authors made to write these accounts.

Samuel L. Milbank
Chairman

Daniel M. Fox
President

Acknowledgments

We acknowledge the assistance of the following individuals who provided invaluable review, comment, and support, making it possible for the public health leaders to tell their stories: Edward L. Baker, Jr., MD, MPH, Director of the Public Health Practice Office, Centers for Disease Control and Prevention; Molly Joel Coye, MD, MPH, Executive Vice President for Strategic Development, Health Desk Corporation, Berkeley; Adele Gonzalez, MPA, Associate Vice-President for Multicultural Affairs and Acting Director for Public Health at the University of North Texas Health Science Center, Fort Worth; Joseph M. Hafey, MPA, Executive Director of the Public Health Institute, Berkeley; Robert K. Ross, MD, Director of the Health and Human Services Agency for the County of San Diego.

Introduction

PUBLIC HEALTH LEADERS NEED TO TELL THEIR STORIES

This book consists of 14 autobiographical chapters about recent events in public health practice in state and local government in the United States. Each author describes how he or she combined scientific knowledge with judgments about how most effectively to apply that knowledge. Each chapter is about the essential elements of public health practice, which are grounded in biomedical and social science and sanctioned by public law. But each also describes the politics of communities and organizations, which are always characterized by conflicts over authority and resources; conflicts that often involve issues of economic competition, social class, culture, and gender.

The editors selected a diverse group of public health practitioners and asked each of them to describe a significant personal experience of leadership. After the authors wrote drafts of their essays, they met to criticize and coach each other. Each of them then wrote another draft that was edited for publication in two issues of the *Journal of Public Health Management and Practice* (3:1 and 3:4). The chapters in this book are, with a few changes, the articles that appeared in the journal.

The authors write from considerable personal experience. They include personal experience. They include persons who have served in senior positions in a dozen states, almost that number of counties, and several major cities. A few have been federal officials; at least three have served as full time faculty members of universities, and one directed health services for an Amerindian nation.

Examples of effective leadership are not easily communicated in the standard rhetoric in which research findings are reported in journals. Leadership is an art, in public health as in any other activity. In every art, method and discipline are preconditions for creativity, courage, timing, and luck. Readers should assume that the authors understand the science and technology that are essential to effective public health practice. These essays are about the art of public health. Hence they are written in the first person, singular, and plural.

The chapters are grouped into five sections. The first consists of three accounts of strategic change in state public health agencies. Charles Mahan tells how he led an effort in Florida to improve the health of women and children by "surrendering control to the locals." Martin P. Wasserman describes the history of a statewide coalition for tobacco control in Maryland from his dual perspective as a county health officer at the beginning of the story and the state's Secretary for Health and Mental Health at the time of writing. Kristine M. Gebbie recounts her experience in building a constituency for public health as health officer for Oregon.

The next stories are about crises; one in Arizona, the other in Texas. Jack Dillenberg, assisted by Douglas Hirano, describes how, as state health officer in Arizona, he confronted a health crisis along the border with Mexico that was generated by environmental pollution. David R. Smith's story about intervention to document and prevent neural tube defects in South Texas combines sophisticated analysis of both science and politics.

Three local health officers write about significant changes in the organization and visibility of public health in their communities. Thomas L. Milne describes how three counties in Washington State achieved a population focus for public health. Paul J. Wiesner tells why and how he led a reorientation of public health activity in DeKalb County, Georgia. Fernando A. Guerra describes changing policy and practice in San Antonio under the accurate title, "The Pope, Hot Pavement, and Public Health."

Three chapters address public health programming, the essential sequel to strategic planning and reorganization. Susan J. Klein tells how the public health agencies of New York State and New York City negotiated partnerships with providers of health services in order to increase the number of individuals receiving directly observed therapy for tuberculosis. Grace G. Eddison describes the challenge of mounting new programs in five counties in Appalachian Eastern Kentucky. Kaye W. Bender writes about the transformation of the state health agency in Mississippi through the development of the "internal consumer."

Three concluding chapters use evidence from the past to raise issues for the future. Lloyd Novick's account of the development of national guidelines for public health practice emphasizes how much easier it is to describe worthwhile innovations than to implement them. Bobbie Berkowitz commends more intense introspection to her colleagues as they assess the politics of public health professionalism. John C. Lewin, reflecting on his career as a physician, health care administrator, public health officer, and medical society executive speculates that anticipating the future may be unrewarding because events seem to have patterns only in retrospect.

Colleagues in every profession inform each other about their range of practical choices in policy and management by telling stories about the past. When such stories are properly told they link theory and method to the contingencies of human experience. The methods of what scholars in the humanities and social sciences call narrative discourse have considerable practical relevance for public health.

The accounts in this book are among the few published stories by active practitioners of public health. We hope these accounts inspire other storytellers, both journalists and autobiographers. Journalists should continue the great tradition of story telling about public health established seven decades ago by Paul de Kruif and carried on in our time by the late Burton Rouché and, recently, by such writers as Laurie Garrett. Practitioners of public health have written engaging memoirs, usually in retirement. The most useful stories about public health leadership have been told to small groups, often in informal settings. We hope this book encourages more leaders to tell their stories.

Lloyd F. Novick
Carol Spain Woltring
Daniel M. Fox

PART I

State Agency Strategies

CHAPTER 1

Surrendering Control
to the Locals

Charles Mahan

Despite the fact that decentralizing decision making is commonly discussed and often praised, few people make the changes to bring it about. In fact, changes in the locus of decision making can be made, yet many top-level leaders really don't want those changes to occur.

A unique leadership challenge I was faced with as Florida's State Health Officer was engineering a shift of policy, program, and financial decision making about the care of mothers and infants from the State Health Office to local coalitions. The key word here is "financial," for I am firmly convinced that if transfer of budgetary authority had not been part of the mandate, far less importance would have been placed on the coalitions and far less positive and negative energy would have been expended on establishing them. In fact, I doubt that many of the coalitions would even exist today, in spite of the legal mandate to have them.

BACKGROUND

In 1974 I was recruited from the University of Minnesota to direct the North Central Florida Maternity and Infant Care Project, a unique collaboration between the University of Florida College of Medicine and 13 surrounding county public health departments. As in Minnesota, I worked closely with state and local public health staff; additionally, my duties required spending two to three days a week caring for patients in various counties. The project was very successful and produced a number of innovations in care for low income populations.

In 1982 the Florida Medical Association and the state health officer asked me to devise a five-year plan to reduce infant mortality in the state. I took a year of sabbatical from the University of Florida and spent it in the state capital completing the plan and educating the legislators about the need for funding. I was asked to continue my responsibilities as director of Maternal and Child Health when the

3

year was up, which I did on an itinerant basis while resuming my academic duties at the University of Florida. In 1987, after successfully completing the five-year plan, I received a large grant from The Robert Wood Johnson Foundation to direct an infant mortality reduction project, entitled the Healthy Futures Program, in the southern states.

I planned to resign as director of Maternal and Child Health to run Healthy Futures when, on the same day, I was called by both the governor's staff and the president of the Florida Medical Association to ask if I would become the new state health officer. I started that job, still a professor "on loan" from the College of Medicine, on January 1, 1988. I relate all of this history because I think it is important for the reader to understand the events that helped develop my "power base," which greatly helped make my leadership efforts successful as State Health Officer.

Many qualities are required for the position of state health officer; among them are leadership skills, mutual respect, professional status, education, and interpersonal skills. Florida has been fortunate, since all state health officers have been handed the power to lead by colleagues who felt that they possessed the attributes listed above. As a result, the title of state health officer comes with an immense amount of good will in our state, which is a great leadership advantage.

I was also fortunate to serve under three governors who, all in their own ways, greatly supported the idea of improving health care for mothers and children. I was brought in as the director of Maternal and Child Health under Democrat Governor Robert Graham, I became state health officer under Republican Governor Robert Martinez, and I was kept in that position by Democrat Governor Lawton Chiles. As a result, I received bipartisan support for public health programs, an important accomplishment considering Florida's rapidly changing politics.

IMPROVING PROGRAMS

Because of the bipartisan political support, we were to make excellent progress in most of our crucial public health programs, especially the Improved Pregnancy Outcome program. When Governor Chiles was elected in 1990, we had a situation in which the governor and his wife, who was deeply committed to keeping mothers and infants healthy, wanted to do something to improve what was already one of our best programs. There were still many improvements to be made, so I welcomed heartily the Chiles's interests. We worked together to craft a bill that would add all the missing elements. When the Florida Healthy Start bill passed into law in 1991, it contained the following:

- Expanded Medicaid eligibility for women earning up to 185 percent of poverty level wages.

- Increased Medicaid payments to maternity care providers to ensure competitive rates.
- Specialist services for high-risk mothers and children at clinics with easier geographic access.
- Mandated risk screening for all pregnant women and all infants at birth.
- State funding for provision of high-risk services, such as Healthy Start services, including nutrition, social work, childbirth education, etc.
- Provision for the development of community Healthy Start Coalitions throughout the state.

HEALTHY START COALITIONS

Responsibilities of the coalitions included the following:

- Assessing health care needs and establishing outcome objectives with guidance from state and national plans.
- Developing a comprehensive resource directory of services available in the coalition's service area.
- Developing a health care services delivery plan that would identify (1) the services required to provide care to priority groups and (2) the unmet needs for services.
- Organizing a local provider network and community organization to implement the delivery of services.
- Developing a method for allocating resources appropriate for the coalition's service area and ensuring that the coalition would be given budget authority by the responsible state or federal agency.
- Developing and implementing a method for evaluating the effectiveness of providers' services compared to outcome objectives.
- Developing a supportive community network within the coalition's service area to ensure that the needs of the priority groups are being met.
- Ensuring that a specific system for maintaining quality health care would be operating within each network provider's organizations.

The vision behind establishing coalitions was that more local control of health care programs would help improve infant outcomes. The coalitions were created as locally focused systems of maternal and child care. Based on need, these systems would improve health outcomes. This outlook focused the coalitions mostly on Medicaid-eligible or potentially Medicaid-eligible people, such as undocumented aliens. Coalition membership included consumers, business people, health professionals, legal and education professionals, political leaders, civic groups, community associations, and advocacy groups. To avoid conflicts of interest, a person could not be a member of a coalition if he received government money for the provision of services related to maternal and child health care.

Duties of the coalitions included:

- A comprehensive community survey of needs for maternal and child health care.
- Development of a comprehensive plan to address those needs.
- Hiring of a full-time coalition manager and support staff. (Each coalition gets $150,000 a year from the state for administration costs.)
- Finding federal, state, or local resources to carry out the plan once it has been approved by experts on maternal and child health care at the State Health Office.
- Monitoring access and quality of services in the local community, and finding different providers if access and quality issues are not addressed satisfactorily.
- Serving as advocates for women and children.
- Developing a public information plan.
- Keeping an up-to-date local resource inventory.
- Helping recruit and retain providers in areas with a shortage of providers.
- Developing close relationships with local and state politicians, in order to educate them on the importance of prevention programs related to maternal and child health care.
- Planning and contracting intensive services for high-risk mothers and infants identified by screening.

Most important, the coalitions were given the power to decide budget policies and priorities for the nonmandated part of all federal and state monies that came to their catchment area for maternal and child health services. This turned out to be a brilliant idea, but for a few years it also turned out to be a strong test of my leadership skills.

COALITION CHALLENGES

The challenges posed by the coalitions began soon after the Healthy Start legislation was signed into law by the governor. I had fully expected that the expansion of Medicaid eligibility for women to 185 percent of poverty income levels and the development and implementation of the screening techniques would be the most difficult parts of the legislation to enact—and technically that was the case. However, early on I started hearing rumblings of discontent about the coalitions from almost every quarter. When boiled down to their essence, most of the growling was about giving up power and control.

At this point, let me say that I personally had to learn firsthand about the value of sharing control and responsibility when leading an organization. Luckily that came to me relatively early, when I was in medical school. I had led a number of organizations before then and, looking back, I held on to power and did not delegate as much as I should have. But there is *nothing* like being president of a group of Type double As in medical school to cure you of *that* leadership style. Those lessons were valuable since they also helped me become an early advocate of team decision making among health care providers. My knowledge also convinced me of the need to share power, knowledge, and responsibility with patients and their families. Because of my experiences, I was able to assume my job as state health officer with populist beliefs and a faith in the abilities of local groups to control their own destinies, even as I joked that my favorite style of leadership was that of benevolent dictatorship.

So when word came back to me—and when you have worked in an organization for 20 years, the word *does* come back—that everyone, from the Secretary of Health and Rehabilitative Services to our staff, to the district administrators, to local health officers, and to local advocacy groups, was in opposition to coalition development, I wasn't too surprised. After all, many people seek these jobs so that they can make things better for citizens, and they believe the way to do that is to work their way up the ladder so that they can have some power and control. Giving power and control away requires a leap of faith. But when a number of the people became hidden barriers, rather like submerged logs in a river, it didn't take long before they were identified.

The problems were reported in various forms: local coalitions complained that the county health officer wouldn't help with the development of the comprehensive plan; one district administrator told his local health officer to make sure that he was elected chair of the coalition so no one outside of the Health and Rehabilitative Services Department would get control; another district administrator complained to the secretary about the content of the local plan, with the result that the secretary objected to family planning being included in it. Additionally, some of our state maternal and child health care staff refused to share knowledge with local coalitions because they wanted to retain control at the state level, and coalition developers complained that state and local health department staffs would not provide the specific data they requested. Staff generally refused to put much time or thought into the coalition issue in the belief that they would not be heard. Because of such opposition, it took a long time before the coalitions were approved and funded. It should not be surprising that those coalitions that met the most resistance from government employees took the longest to develop; some of them came about a full two years after the first were approved.

To be fair, some barriers to coalition development were thrown up by the local developers themselves. Unfortunately, some hired administrators spent their time asking for more state money to build more administrative capacity rather than making progress toward coalition goals. Others became angry because the staff could not provide data sets. Many people were also hampered by little or no understanding of basic statistics.

As I think about the problems presented above, I realize the issues do not sound as compelling as having to deal with, say, terrorists poisoning the New York City water supply. However, they received my attention for a couple of reasons. First, most of these barriers were being erected by friends and colleagues, not to torment me, but because they didn't believe in local coalitions having autonomy. I had to solve these problems, but in such a way that I kept a close and effective working relationship with everyone involved, primarily so that I could depend on their help with the myriad other public health issues, present and future. Second, the governor and his wife were, and still are, deeply interested in the subject of maternal and child health care and know more about the medical details of such care than do most doctors. I have joked that the governor called me every day to inquire about changes in the infant mortality rate, but that after I gave him a brief lecture on basic statistics, he only called me every other day. (In fact, he did ask, and frequently.) Additionally, Governor Chiles visited developing coalitions whenever he could. So I certainly felt great pressure to make the Healthy Start program and its components successful. Of course, it didn't hurt that it was also one of my own major areas of interest.

DEVELOPING SOLUTIONS

I did not sit down and think out an overall strategy to solve these problems, especially since they presented themselves piecemeal over a period of about a year and a half. First, I dealt with threats perceived by the state health officer's maternal and child health care staff. These were superb professionals, most of whom I had worked with for almost 10 years. They had seen the programs they helped direct from the state level reap great returns in reduction of infant deaths, and they felt comfortable in continuing those same efforts. I reminded staff that external consultants thought we had reduced our overall infant mortality rate by such a large amount that we had probably effected as much change as we could in reducing "easier to solve" causes of infant mortality. Now we needed to attack the hard-core problems, such as cocaine use, which were not statewide but localized in specific areas and communities.

This idea was accepted, but a bigger issue came up, namely, that the state staff was overwhelmed with devising screening instruments and meeting the deadlines for the statewide screening of close to 400,000 mothers and infants. Staff felt they had neither the time nor patience to deal with the constant needs of the local people developing the coalitions. To solve this problem, I contacted the state director of Medicaid, and we worked out a way of jointly funding contracts with faculty and staff of the University of South Florida College of Public Health. Our goals were to deal directly with development problems of the coalitions and to serve as an intermediary between the local coalitions and the state health officer's maternal and child health care staff. The contract with the university was called Healthy Beginnings. It was considered an expansion of early efforts to evaluate the Improved Pregnancy Outcome Program and to enlarge the Medicaid program.

Healthy Start encompassed many activities. Developing coalitions were assisted with applications for full coalition status and funding. The coalitions were also helped with recruiting the required mix of people onto the board. Consultations were offered on the development of local coalition bylaws and policies. Healthy Start rules and regulations were interpreted so that legislative intent was met. Staff were introduced to community health assessment methodologies such as PATCH (Planned Approach to Community Health) and APEX-PH (Assessment Protocol for Excellence in Public Health) and were assisted in working the results into an action plan that would receive consensus support from coalition members. The program additionally acted as an intermediary to resolve disputes and strengthen working relationships with public health entities from the state to the local level.

The University of South Florida's research files and resources were used to help coalitions identify potential funders for some of their local efforts. Coalitions developed skills in conflict resolution, consensus building, and team building. Healthy Beginnings also helped structure evaluations of local providers of health care services and administrative procedures. Coalitions were assisted in understanding the delivery of health care, social service, and economic benefits services. Coalitions were taught about the rapid changes occurring in the health care delivery system, such as the development of Medicaid managed care and health maintenance organizations.

Coalitions were also assisted in understanding the maze of funding sources for maternal and child health care, including Medicaid, private insurance, Improved Pregnancy Outcome, Title V, and Healthy Start. Those services not funded by anyone were also delineated. Other activities included working with coalitions to access data tools and analysis from the State Health Office, State Medicaid Office, county health units, and the College of Public Health; helping develop, support, and renew local coalition leadership; assisting with community-based planning and policy making; and convening maternal and child health care advocates, state agencies, and coalition representatives on a regular basis to share solutions and plan improvements.

Fortunately, the College of Public Health was able to have a point person for this contract, a woman who was a superb leader, a well-known staff person highly respected by all players throughout the state, and a tireless worker who had labored for years to make our efforts succeed.

Next, I had to deal with 15 district administrators, who ignored almost everything that had to do with health and did not support program efforts such as outposting workers in health departments to help pregnant women fulfill eligibility requirements for services. As I mentioned before, there were those who were determined to keep control of the coalitions rather than turn power over. First, I addressed district administrators from around the state at one of their monthly meetings, presenting the reasons for having local coalitions. I explained that the coalitions would help marshal extra local resources, including money and volunteers, would provide local political support for our programs, and so on. Unfortunately, my words did not reach the audience, and so, in a further effort, I had coalition members in each district meet personally with each of the district administrators, and that had some slight success.

Finally, I had to resort to saying "Big Guy and Mrs. Big Guy want this to happen!" Every communication sent to and received from the governor about and from the coalitions was copied and distributed among the district administrators. The reports I gave to the district administrators at their meetings were placed first, not last, on their agendas, and the governor's active involvement and interest in the coalitions were heavily emphasized. Finally, I asked the coalition developers in the most recalcitrant districts to invite the governor to one of their functions. When he appeared at those, so did the local district administrator, who was newly briefed on the details of Healthy Start and coalitions by staff. In the end, the district administrators were greatly impressed with the governor's real interest in the coalitions, and all of them came to support the changes.

There was a bizarre situation in which the Secretary of Health and Rehabilitative Services sided with the local district administrator against the local coalition and against the local health officer when local staff wanted to strengthen and expand local family planning efforts to prevent unintended pregnancies (one of the most effective methods to lower infant mortality and morbidity). Although the secretary was strongly against family planning for personal religious reasons, he had been able to suppress his feelings up to this point. But when he sided with the district administrator, I went to discuss the issue with him, and he stood firm in his opposition. As we explored the problem further, he revealed that he really did not want local groups deciding the destiny of his agency, *especially* if they were going to address issues he did not agree with. We argued about this, but he remained resolute.

I shared this conversation with group members advocating family planning, only to find out that they had called me after they had already expressed concern to the governor's office about the issue. Luckily that week I was flying with the governor and his wife to a coalition meeting. I had prepared a presentation on the importance of family planning for reducing infant mortality, a concept they already generally supported, and had a full hour alone with them to discuss the issue.

By the time we landed, the governor and his wife agreed that the coalitions should make family planning a priority issue. Additionally, the governor promised to emphasize his decision to the secretary. I was then able to send a letter to all coalitions and district administrators stating that the governor had agreed that all coalitions should target family planning as one of their top issues.

Essentially the same methods that were used with the district administrators were used to educate local health officers to get their cooperation on and input about the development of local coalitions. My observation was that the roughly 25 percent of local health officers who resisted the development of coalitions were the same people who were the weakest at working cooperatively with their communities. After I had bombarded the district administrators with information about the governor's keen interest in the program, most of them eventually gave in. However, giving power to local coalitions resulted in constant local scrutiny of all players in the field. The close examination led to such dissatisfaction in certain areas that we had to replace three health officers.

Dealing with coalition complaints and leadership problems proved a time-consuming, delicate process. The state health officer's staff and Medicaid staff expended much time and effort teaching coalitions what data were even possible to access. Much time was also spent educating coalitions on basic statistics, statistical significance, and even why they really should not want or need certain data they had requested. My role in this process was to attend many of the more problematic meetings to back up our staff and to ensure that the coalition decision-makers would show up, pay attention, and come to a consensus.

Leadership problems in coalitions were much harder to deal with because of the mandate to let the local coalitions control their own destinies. However, in some instances people hired to manage coalitions were inept, and boards had to be counseled that funding from the state might have to be held back until these persons were dealt with. There was a further problem: Board presidents were in constant conflict with state staff. My role in mediating all these issues, which I recognized as growing pains of fledgling organizations, was to meet regularly with the Healthy Start and Healthy Beginnings staffs and offer guidance and support. Again I was fortunate that the leaders of these two groups were totally dedicated people who were highly effective in dealing with these problems.

POSITIVE OUTCOMES

All our efforts were finally successful, and by the end of 1993, Florida was the only state with a complete capacity for community-based planning and resource allocation in maternal and child health care. Thirty Healthy Start coalitions had been established, serving all 67 counties. Local coalitions became the focus for all maternal and child health care assessment and assurance functions for the 30 communities, with local health departments as partners. Local resources marshaled 2,250 volunteers, who gave more than 50,000 hours of service and raised millions of local dollars in cash and in-kind services. The data system documenting maternal and child health care improved to become the best in the country, enabling RAND to do a detailed study on the effects of expansion of Medicaid coverage in the state. Coalitions began participating in the unique statewide program for the improvement of public health, and this led to the establishment of nine fetal and infant mortality review projects across the state, with more being developed.

The coalitions closely watched hospitals with low completion rates for Healthy Start screening forms, as well as those institutions that neglected to perform voluntary tubal interruptions postpartum. Ultimately the coalitions wished to develop interview processes to help evaluate the quality of care given by local managed care organizations. Other positive outcomes included the creation of strong ties with the private sector, especially private physicians, and helping infuse new energy and authority into traditional advocacy groups for mother and child health care, which included childbirth educators, the March of Dimes organization, and the state perinatal association. The Healthy Start coalitions have stimulated other public-private partnership activity, involving local groups such as the Kiwanis organization, which supports immunizations; the Cancer Society, which backs anti-smoking coalitions; and others.

Most important, mother and child health care has improved to a point where care is often better for poor women than care received by women from the upper-income bracket in the same community. Healthy Start recipients generally indicate high satisfaction with their care. Thanks to the work of the coalitions, all pregnant women in Florida now receive prenatal care, and it looks as if the state will reach the national infant mortality goal of 7 per 1,000 live births two or three years before the year 2000.

OBSERVATIONS

I can't think of any negative consequences resulting from the establishment of the coalitions. Reflecting on lessons learned from this case, I can make a few observations. Some people who clamor for leadership responsibility find they really don't want it when they finally get it. This was seen in the few coalition leaders who didn't last long.

Efforts should be made to study ways to encourage state governments to restructure their state health officer positions into nonpolitical, long-tenure posts (as occurs in Britain) by focusing on the health and science aspects of the position. Also, the need for stable leadership would foster the development and maintenance of long-term programs and interventions. Statewide leaders need to constantly determine which functions are most effectively done at the local versus the state level by experimenting with innovative local initiatives.

Effective leadership usually involves relinquishing power or sharing power with colleagues at many levels. This helps gain trust and authority for the leader. Also, sharing "money power"—the power to make financial rather than just philosophical decisions—with coalitions is an important step to let them know you are serious about their work. I strongly believe this will keep the coalitions functioning for many years.

"Walking-around management" is very effective, even if it requires traveling across an entire state. In addition, in public health, one of the most effective leadership tools, is good science, based on good scholarship and good data, presented in a simple educational format.

Finally, work steadily toward your goals. If reducing infant mortality is the goal, then every leadership challenge is best met with a focus on infant mortality, rather than on process issues such as personnel, funding, space, etc. Constantly reminding colleagues of the goals the group is after is the best way to have everyone working toward a common purpose.

Our next governor may be primarily interested in transportation or tourism, not mothers and infants. Even if such a change in emphasis occurs, I feel confident that the leadership efforts invested in the Healthy Start coalitions will protect and improve those services for a long time after the current governor and I are gone.

CHAPTER 2

Building a Statewide Coalition for Tobacco Control, 1993–Present

Martin P. Wasserman

For over 40 years either Maryland, Delaware, or the District of Columbia has led the nation in deaths from cancer. In Maryland, lung cancer is responsible for the greatest number of cancer deaths; because most cases of lung cancer result from long-term tobacco use, lung cancer is considered easily preventable through appropriate interventions.

In 1991, the Maryland Cancer Consortium—a group of researchers, community leaders, and policy makers—identified priorities and came up with strategies to reduce and prevent lung, breast, and cervical cancers (Maryland Cancer Control Plan, Maryland Cancer Consortium, January 1991). The authors of the Maryland Cancer Control Plan identified tobacco use as the primary risk factor contributing to cancer mortality in Maryland. The Plan recommended several strategies to reduce tobacco use, including policy changes, mass media advertising, and educational interventions.

Although individuals and many interest groups were eager to join forces lowering tobacco use so as to erase the stigma of being the state with the greatest number of deaths from cancer, Maryland is also a tobacco-growing state. Many people who support the idea of cancer prevention were skeptical whether the Cancer Control Plan could be implemented.

By the spring of 1992, many significant policy changes were taking place. Despite litigation, the towns of Bowie and Takoma Park and Montgomery County, Maryland, were attempting to severely limit placement of tobacco vending machines. A cigarette excise tax increase, strongly supported by the governor's Cancer Council, was passed. Some communities and counties had passed ordinances restricting smoking in public places. Governor William Donald Schaefer issued an executive order requiring that state buildings be smoke free, becoming one of the first governors in the United States to take this action. The State Health Department began advocating policy change as an accompaniment to media and educational interventions in order to reduce access of young persons to tobacco products and protect the general population in public places.

A major obstacle, however, was the lack of grassroots support for policy and legislative change. A broad-based statewide coalition made up of advocates and community organizations was needed.

A CALL TO ACTION

Having recently been elected President of the Local Health Officers Association in Maryland, I was becoming more aware of relationships between state and local government. My experience was teaching me how to make good public health policy on a statewide basis without preventing local governments from enacting more stringent legislation. Because of our state's problems with cancer, I concluded that statewide action on tobacco control was needed and would require, first and foremost, a gathering of all appropriate players involved in reducing the cancer rate.

Earlier in the year, because of a past relationship with Irene Polin, wife of Abe Polin, the owner of the Washington Bullets—we both served on the Secretary of Health and Human Services's Council on Disease Prevention and Health Promotion—I had been asked to make recommendations for a healthy lifestyle for the wives of the Washington Bullets basketball players. I suggested an approach that included exercise and no tobacco use, and I urged the wives to include their husbands in this effort.

Unfortunately, for a variety of reasons, this project was never begun, remaining merely an unexecuted plan. But another opportunity was created when the chairperson of the Cancer Summit Program, Connie Unseld, the wife of the Washington Bullets basketball coach, received a last minute cancellation from one of her scheduled speakers. The emphasis of that year's summit was on tobacco-related malignancies and, remembering my interest in the subject, she asked me if I would be willing to speak as a replacement. When I learned of the diverse backgrounds of those attending the summit, I realized that the summit represented an opportunity for me to create an action-oriented coalition from the membership who would be present, and so I accepted the invitation to speak. During the speech, I challenged this group of approximately 300 government officials, physicians, academicians, community health workers, elected officials, and tobacco control advocates to take the information being discussed at the summit and convert it to action, to actually *do* something. My objective was to gather the energy of all the players in Maryland interested in controlling cancer; our goal was to work toward and make Maryland the new leader in tobacco control.

I invited those individuals who were truly interested in putting their ideas into action to meet within the month, on June 9, 1993, at the offices of the state medical society. The purpose of the meeting would be to form a coalition, determine a proactive and inclusive strategy, and assist the governor in developing comprehensive anti-tobacco legislation. The speech was well received, and on June 9th, nearly 60 people, including the state's attorney general, arrived at the meeting. This, in effect, was the first meeting of our group, entitled Smoke Free Maryland: A Coalition for Tobacco Control. What was critical, I believe, was the emphasis on bringing the group together to form its own agenda rather than on implementing a predetermined plan of action. We focused on process and believed it would determine the appropriate outcome.

POLITICAL TERRAIN

Governor Schaefer was embarrassed by the negative publicity Maryland was receiving because of its high ranking nationwide in cancer mortality. He decided to attempt lowering Maryland's cancer rate by focusing on prevention and promoting healthy lifestyles, particularly for young people. Although he did not declare open warfare on the tobacco industry, he had no particular allegiance to it. Schaefer successfully introduced legislation to increase the excise tax on cigarettes and restrict minors' access to tobacco. He also introduced a ban on use of tobacco products in the worksite and supported a school bylaw change to prohibit the use of tobacco products on all school property. Finally, by executive order the governor banned the use of tobacco products in state office buildings and eliminated tobacco advertising on state-owned transit vehicles (Maryland Executive Order 0101.1992.20). However, the tobacco industry fought back, succeeding in using the courts to block the worksite smoking regulation and in preventing local jurisdictions from passing stronger tobacco vending machine restrictions than the state had passed.

At that time, there were only a few advocates for tobacco control in the state legislature. This group consisted mainly of a small number of women legislators and people with health care backgrounds or a special interest in public health. Some legislators were smokers, and a few owned bars or other small businesses. These individuals did not want the government to intervene in their lives or businesses by preventing tobacco use. Despite the governor's executive order banning smoking in government buildings, smoking was permitted in the legislative chambers, hearing rooms, and offices. Perhaps most important, election campaigns were heavily financed by organizations with strong links to the tobacco industry. In fact, the most visible and indeed the most popular campaign financier was the Tobacco Institute's lobbyist, Bruce Bereano. The legislature also had many representatives with personal or constituent relationships to the industry. Politically, therefore, tobacco control was considered "a tough sell" in the house and senate of Maryland's legislature.

At the center of the tobacco control debate is the issue of state versus local control of tobacco policies. A handful of people had fought hard to have local governing bodies, like the Montgomery County Council, whose members represent Maryland's largest and most liberal jurisdiction, pass a policy forbidding smoking in enclosed public places (Montgomery County Council Bill 27–87, 1987). Although this local law passed while I was the Montgomery County Health Officer, some members of the group felt that I had not gone far enough in supporting their recommendations. I believed that I had done what was possible and practical at the time. Because I viewed some elements of the plan as too extreme for the council to accept, I did not extend my complete support for the plan as the group originally conceived it. At the state level, these activists were most interested in passing a law guaranteeing local governments the right to pass laws that were more restrictive than the state's in preventing tobacco use. This was referred to as the "preemption issue."

The voluntary organizations in our state, such as the Lung Association, the Cancer Society, and the Heart Association were very active in efforts limiting tobacco use. Although they were in favor of local jurisdictions making headway on control of tobacco use, they had spent years building relationships in the state legislature and were interested in passing statewide legislation that would restrict minors' access to tobacco. Because of their interest in passing statewide legislation, they were not as interested in passing a law that would increase local government's power to control tobacco use beyond that of the state's power, viewing that element of the legislation as a potential barrier to successful passage of their plan. If the local preemption protection was not written into law, then each local jurisdiction would have to develop specific state legislation for each bill controlling tobacco. But this situation would make it very difficult for the statewide bills to pass. Given those circumstances, advocates of tobacco control were divided about what to do, and indeed those who opposed tobacco control encouraged them to argue over their differences, thereby immobilizing the effort.

The tobacco industry had both overt and covert supporters in the Maryland legislature. They had been in control for so long that conventional wisdom assumed that statewide tobacco control victories would be either impossible or small at best. Given the tobacco industry's long-standing successful relationship with the Maryland legislature and the stature of their primary lobbyist, it did not feel threatened by either the local tobacco control activists or the do-good enthusiasts from the voluntary organizations. The industry's objectives were to keep their opponents fighting among themselves and to focus most of their energies at the state level, where they had the most influence. This strategy allowed the tobacco industry to avoid costly battles at the local level.

The attorney general and his office had been very supportive of anti-tobacco efforts, particularly in the areas of restricting billboard advertising, but up until this time had not taken a highly visible position in the area of tobacco control initiatives. The attorney general would attend the first meeting of the coalition and pledge his personal support and that of his office to reducing tobacco's harmful effects in the state of Maryland.

The Maryland State Medical Society (Med-Chi) had just begun to compete for grants and take on their own projects oriented toward improving health. Although they had a long history of being involved with the state legislature, they were perceived primarily as supporting the financial interests of physicians and being less involved in issues relating to the public's health. At the time of the first meeting of the coalition, I was serving as Chairman of their Public Health Committee. The society had made tobacco control a priority on its legislative agenda and the President of Med-Chi offered the organization as a resource and a facilitator of anti-tobacco efforts and was personally very supportive on this issue.

After an explosion ignited by a cigarette killed three school maintenance workers, the Secretary of Licensing and Regulation asked the Maryland Occupational Safety and Health (MOSH) Advisory Board to consider regulations banning smoking in enclosed workplaces. The board pursued the cause on the scientific evidence that smoking and secondhand smoke was a danger to health. During the 1993 legislative session, the Local Health Officers' Association had been successful in passing a bill restoring some of the funding for local health departments previously eliminated by the governor. This effort represented the debut of this group of local public health officials on the state legislative scene and they were excited by their success. Fresh from victory, the Local Health Officers' Association, supportive of statewide action for tobacco control, was eager to participate in group efforts. Since Maryland has a health officer heading a local health department in each of its 24 jurisdictions, communication and contact with the health department at the local level was easily achieved. Indeed, Maryland was the first state in the country to have appointed health officers in each county and the city of Baltimore and so had the structural capability for active, concerted, and consolidated activity on a statewide basis.

Leading oncologists from the Johns Hopkins School of Medicine and the University of Maryland served on the governor's Cancer Council. Their involvement ensured that the academic medical institutions were political participants in this effort. In addition, in 1991, the Johns Hopkins School of Public Health had entered into a collaborative relationship with the Local Health Officers' Association through the Johns Hopkins Health Program Alliance. This relationship involved university faculty in public health initiatives and helped provide additional support to tobacco control.

PRINCIPLE-CENTERED STRATEGIES

At the first meeting in June of 1993, the group discussed its reason for being, giving members an opportunity to speak and state their particular area of focus. The next efforts involved reviewing the previous year's legislation and formulating a set of principles to guide the organization. The following principles were adopted by the group at its meeting on July 28, 1993.

1. Children should be protected by enforcement of laws against selling tobacco to minors. This must include increasing fines and mandating eventual suspension and revocation of licenses for those who repeatedly sell tobacco to minors.
2. Children should be protected by limiting the placement of tobacco vending machines.
3. Employees should be protected by law in their right to a smoke-free work environment.
4. The public should be protected by making enclosed public places free of environmental tobacco smoke.
5. The state should not preempt counties and municipalities from enacting stronger legislation.
6. The state should increase taxes on all tobacco products.

Four subcommittee work groups were created with the following purposes: to draft legislation; to support media/marketing activities; to involve the community at the grassroots level; and to provide alternatives to legislation activities, such as enforcement and regulation.

The grassroots work group immediately began to identify county coordinators for each jurisdiction. Most coordinators were local health officers, or local health department personnel, or known tobacco control activists from the community. A private physician volunteered to coordinate the coordinators and established a phone and fax tree system for rapid communication and dissemination of information. Members of the grassroots committee began meeting with legislators during the summer and early fall, and brought with them the county coordinators from the legislator's home jurisdiction to focus attention on tobacco control as an issue of constituent concern.

While local legislative discussion and education were being pursued, the group set out to identify community support organizations to sign up in support of controlling tobacco use. By the fall of 1993, there was a comprehensive list of about 20 organizations that had endorsed the group's principles, including health care provider organizations, youth advocacy organizations, private voluntary organizations, university medical schools, the Parent Teacher Association, public health associations, and others.

The membership of the legislation-drafting work group included an attorney who worked for the state medical society. His expertise with the law, coupled with the experience of some of the activists, enabled the work group to map out a sophisticated legislative strategy. By December 1993, the work group had developed draft bills to restrict minors' access to tobacco products and limit the locations where vending machines could be placed in the state. These bills were ultimately presented to Governor Schaefer with the hope that they would be introduced as his own. The work group also recommended that the administration support antipreemption legislation and prohibit smoking in designated indoor public places.

The real work as the leader of the coalition centered around the issue of whether the coalition as a group should support antipreemption legislation. Such legislation, if passed by the General Assembly, would permit localities to enact stricter laws and regulations governing the sale of tobacco products and restriction of smoking in public places than those provided by state law. To those members of the coalition who had been successful in restricting smoking and sale of tobacco at the local level, this was crucial to their attempts to limit tobacco use. However, it seemed a risky political fight to those of us who wanted to protect every Maryland citizen, since many legislators opposed the local measure but stated they would support a statewide bill. We knew that in many Maryland jurisdictions nothing would be accomplished through local political action, and so we believed a statewide effort would be required for any restriction in tobacco use.

At the coalition meeting held in December of 1993, prior to the start of the legislative session in January, the work group drafting legislation presented the draft bills to the coalition. Nelson Sabatini, the Maryland Secretary of Health, came to the meeting on behalf of the governor and thanked the coalition for the work done on drafting the legislation. He then stated that while each of the coalition's bills limiting minors' access to tobacco had a clause against preemption legislation in them, the governor had decided that the preemption issue should be considered on its own. Consequently, in the administration's bills the two bills limiting minors' access to tobacco would be considered on their own, and a separate bill spelling out the issue of restricting preemptive legislation would also be introduced by the governor.

Separating the bills caused considerable disruption among coalition members. Although I personally supported this approach, I did my best to respond to the position of each coalition member at the meeting so as to keep us all focused and together. Many members stated their opinion that the governor, who had been a strong, previous advocate for preemption on a local level was "selling out" to the tobacco industry by decoupling the issues. I knew that much of the coalition's strength came from its close relationship and cooperative working relationship with the state health department and the governor and I did not want to sacrifice that. Nevertheless, in support of the desire of our members, as convener of the coalition, I agreed to write a letter to the governor expressing our desire that he leave the language against preemption legislation in the minors' access bills. We also asked that he introduce a stand-alone bill against such legislation. As an alternative, we would introduce our own independent legislation, something that eventually did happen.

The coalition's strategy was to find sponsors for the bills drafted by the coalition and support those. If a member of the coalition testified on behalf of the coalition, he or she would have to support the governor's position but say that the coalition felt that the intent of the bill would be strengthened by adding the antipreemption clause. This took a lot of tough negotiating with the growing group of coalition members, who at this point numbered about 30 regular attendees, and there were some tense moments during that legislative session when the activists pressed their case more aggressively than the voluntary agencies representing the state's cancer society, heart and lung associations, and other coalition members wanted them to. Toward the end of the legislative session, the activists were not invited to coalition meetings.

Eventually we came out of the session with comprehensive legislation limiting minors' access to tobacco, but the legislation did not include the antipreemption clause. The bill signed into law was somewhat of a mixed blessing, for although it increased the fines for selling cigarettes to minors, it made it a civil offense for minors to buy or possess tobacco products. Minors committing such an infraction could be fined or ordered to attend smoking cessation classes (punishing minors who purchased tobacco was the tobacco industry's idea). This provision was part of a deal made with the voluntaries long before the session started.

The tobacco lobby was successful in fighting off a cigarette tax increase, a bill that was very important to the governor. The bill started out as a tax increase of 25 cents per pack. Later, the bill was amended to require that the state tax increase to 30 percent of the amount of any raise in federal tax. This was not acceptable to legislative leadership and was never brought up for a vote in the state senate.

FUNDING FOR THE COALITION: ROBERT WOOD JOHNSON

Before the coalition was created, the Maryland Department of Health and Mental Hygiene launched an education campaign in 1992, which included development of school-based curricula for controlling tobacco use, community grants, and a media campaign focusing on the effects of secondhand smoke and the prevention of smoking initiation among school-aged youth. In December 1993, representatives of the health department along with other coalition members began to put together an application for a grant of $1 million in matching funds for the coalition from the Robert Wood Johnson Foundation's "Smokeless States" initiative.

ANOTHER AVENUE FOR CHANGE: STATE REGULATION OF SMOKING IN THE WORKPLACE

In April 1994, the MOSH board issued regulations banning smoking in the workplace, including bars and restaurants, in response to the death of three school maintenance workers from an explosion (Maryland Registered Code [COMAR] Title 09 Dept. of Licensing and Regulation, 12.23.01-05 [1995]). Then in May, the legislative committee that reviews regulations heard the proposed changes after which it sent a letter to the governor stating that the legislature wanted to look over the regulations. The controversy forced the issue back into the legislative arena. A compromise was struck—the ban excludes bars and the bar area of restaurants—and the regulations went into effect in March of 1995.

LESSONS

In December 1994, the newly elected Governor Parris Glendening appointed me Maryland's Secretary for Health and Mental Hygiene. My political education has now entered its latest phase. The events described previously, like many others in my career, are part of my cumulative and continuing education in the practice as well as the ideals of public health. Of particular value during this process was my building consensus by working with a variety of constituencies. The strategies developed to move the process forward and gain the respect of the legislature would provide early personal credibility to me as I began my role as Secretary. Leading such a varied group of individuals and keeping them "on track" was a tremendous experience for the many challenges subsequently faced. Working with a group to determine just how far one could go on an issue of strong political advocacy taught me much about the political process. Each lesson built upon the previous one, and together have provided me with many additional skills and tools to use in support of the public's health in my current role.

CHAPTER 3

Building a Constituency for Public Health

Kristine M. Gebbie

Many public health professionals believe they lack the powerful constituency that will push for improved funding and visibility, in contrast to the many groups that rally to support a hospital threatened with closure or to support an emerging, promising, but unfunded medical procedure. In fact, powerful groups that have frequent contact with public health agencies too often become critics of them: Businesses subject to public health regulation intended to control environmental threats or to assure the quality of health-related services are often found lobbying against the public health structure.

Concerned about this apparent lack of support, public health leaders have become aware that they need to build a constituency. They seek groups to speak on behalf of public health and population-based approaches to health improvement. The relatively new Partnership for Prevention organization represents a national coalition-building effort; Public Health Week activities each April include state and local outreach. Public health leaders also want some groups to support specific agencies in specific areas of interest, such as annual budget debates or legislative work.

As a public health director, I have also experienced those needs for support, and I have attempted to build constituencies that would be there when needed. This case study is based on my 11 years as head of the Health Division, Oregon Department of Human Resources, the agency responsible for preserving and protecting the health of all Oregonians. The study describes building the components of a constituency for public health, specifically for the state public health agency in Oregon, an effort that I believe is closely related to building a more generic advocacy for the health of the public of the state.

THE CASE OF OREGON

In 1978, I arrived in Portland to become head of the state's public health agency. In the approximately six years since the state had merged its board of health, along with seven other agencies, into the Department of Human Resources, the Health Division had experienced five administrators in quick succession, the longest tenured of whom had stayed in office for just over 18 months. None of the administrators had previous health-related clinical or management experience. The general expectation of staff was that administrators would continue to come and go, and that the best course of action was to keep your head down, perform your job very quietly, and hope no one would ever notice you.

Both state and local public health staff believed that these administrators were not to be trusted because they would sacrifice good public health for political peace, and therefore difficult public health decisions were to be kept away from the top staff of the agency. Failure to build a constituency for public health in the state could well make this expectation real. And if that state of affairs continued, there would be little interest in investing new resources in the Health Division, little public support in the case of conflict, and a decreasing likelihood that the legislature would strengthen the capacity of the division to respond to threats to the health of Oregonians.

Complicating any efforts at constituency building were three environmental factors: the nature of being a chief public health official within an umbrella agency, the legacy of relationships (not always positive) between the state and local public health agencies, and the economic climate in Oregon at that time. With regard to the structure of state government, it is generally accepted by public health officials that it is better to be an independent cabinet appointee (preferably with the political cushion of a board of health) than to report through someone to the governor. In Oregon, during the time I was there, Department of Human Resources division administrators worked directly with the governor, attending cabinet meetings with the Department of Human Resources director and working directly with other executive branch agencies, albeit always in collaboration with the department as a whole.

The significant negative, in my experience, was the distinctly different world view of the other agencies of the department and its central management staff. Other constituencies were very specific, associated with a relatively small proportion of the state's population: Only a limited number of persons were on public assistance, in a state mental hospital or prison, or on the unemployment rolls at any one time. The common language of "caseload" and "stakeholder" assumed a very different meaning when applied to the Health Division, for which the entire state population was the "client" all of the time.

After creation of the Department of Human Resources, the local health departments had never developed a strong relationship with any of the Health Division

administrators, concentrating instead on fairly independent projects (such as establishing standards for local health department performance) and on relationships
with individual programs within the Health Division. To the extent that the local
health departments could speak with one voice, they represented public health in
the state, and to the extent that they built up their most important constituency—
local elected officials—they could command a good deal of attention from the
legislature or other decision makers. Any effort by the Health Division to build a
constituency that might be interested in statewide concerns and that did not fully
support the individual autonomy of local public health efforts was seen as a potential threat and could trigger a high level of opposition.

Finally, Oregon entered the economic downturn of the early 1980s earlier, and
more severely, than many other states. A dramatic drop in timber sales and timber-
related employment, with associated losses in public revenue, meant that budget
cutting and staff layoffs became the order of the day. This was exacerbated, following Reagan's election to the presidency, by the introduction of block grants
and what was termed the "new federalism," which meant state agencies had to
take responsibility for making cuts in programs and resources actually stemming
from federal decisions. Building a constituency when resources are shrinking is
extremely difficult, because it takes a long-term perspective and a high level of
confidence to step back from individual interests to consider a more general good.
It would have done public health no good to stimulate individual constituencies
that then publicly competed with one another for shrinking resources. I had to look
for support for the whole.

There were several strong advantages I enjoyed as a player new to a state need-
ing to build public health constituencies. The first was the apprenticeship in management that I had served in my previous employment as an assistant director in a
university medical center. My supervisor there was a strong member of the medical center management team, with an outcome-oriented approach that required
stating and then working to achieve goals. I had been taught to identify internal
and external constituencies and then work with them to fulfill my share of the
organization's goals. Second, I joined a strong leadership team in Oregon, in a
department that at that time was invested in management development. Soon after
arriving in the state, I was able to spend a week with other senior managers under
the tutelage of an expert in organizational development. The role of stakeholders
and constituencies was a significant portion of the material taught, and I had the
opportunity to reflect on what needed to be done.

Within six months of my arrival, I had made two management decisions, one
regarding a personnel matter, the other a public health regulatory issue that became an issue in which the media were strongly interested. The public response
reinforced my awareness of the need to have a constituency that understood public
health, the role of the state's public health agency, and me as its leader. Finally,

because of my training and experience in health systems, community development, and nursing, I was perceived as a professional appointee, rather than a political one. The public and the staff believed that I could be trusted and should be supported because I would understand the public health rationale for decisions and would support public health in the face of political pressures.

DEFINING THE MISSION AND THE CASELOAD

The efforts devoted to building the internal constituency included many familiar in management development: involving management staff in writing an agency mission statement; creating and sustaining an agencywide new employee orientation; and devoting careful attention to ensure that internal documents and materials leaving the agency were consistent in framework and language. I also attempted to regularly visit agency staff in their workplaces, providing them an opportunity to show off new projects or activities; at the same time, I was becoming familiar with the day-to-day work environment. While this was helpful, hindsight suggested that I did not do enough in the first year, partly because of the time I committed to learning about the local health departments, as discussed later.

Document development had particular importance in building the department's central staff as a potential constituency for the division. Although, through experience, budget and policy staff at the Department of Human Resources expected the Health Division to provide uncoordinated and often inconsistent materials, this was tolerated because it was the smallest division in staff and budget, and so the problems were seen as relatively unimportant. The division followed standardized formats, making no attempt to clarify how such formats might distort the case of public health. For example, in answering the question of caseload served, the division might list the number of epidemiologic investigations rather than acknowledge that all Oregonians were served by the prompt investigation and check of food- or water-borne disease outbreaks. There was no systematic way to identify the staff, budget, or workload of the local public health agency partners in routine reports. It was a major step when I was able to get agreement that the service offered by the Health Division was to support local public health through laboratory, epidemiology, public health nursing, and sanitarian consultation. The alternative—describing those services as the responsibility of the central administration—was shelved.

This process extended to using the biennial budget development process as a major communications tool. Historically, most attention had been given to the numbers, with individual programs writing required narratives independently. After one legislative cycle under this system, I made the decision that we needed a coherent narrative that would tie together all budget parts and that would clearly identify priorities and decisions. This meant increasing management time in collective budget work. We wanted to make certain that program intersections were identified and that the highest priority goals were consistently highlighted. An individual with strong writing skills completely rewrote the entire document to deliver a single message. Doing this was painful; not all programs were described as most critical to keeping the state healthy! But despite the pains, organizational strength was built as staff learned to work as a team and as the department and legislature learned that they could expect consistency across the division. A consistent building toward priorities requires time.

An interrelated development was the long-term effort to strengthen the Health Division's information capacity. While there had been a vital records program for three-quarters of a century, and while epidemiology reports were published regularly, it was not unusual for state or local program decisions to be based on disease or health status reports two years old or more. And there was no assurance that relevant health information was getting to health professionals or the public in a timely and useful manner. To do so would require the upgrading of an information-processing capacity. Over several budget cycles, funds were allocated for upgrading computer capacity, health statistics and epidemiology were combined into a new health status monitoring unit, and the publication of timely information in readily accessible form was made a priority. This increased media use of our information, and those institutions that were able to make use of the improved information, including health professional associations, academic centers, and local health departments, became greater advocates of public health.

Speaking with one voice was also associated with increasing the public visibility of the division, primarily through the administrator's media presence. Some of this was inadvertent, springing from the negative publicity surrounding the two early decisions mentioned above. The first was about the abrupt termination of two long-time staff members due to mismanagement of income from the sale of vital records.

I had originally supported the action, basing my decision on a staff recommendation without fully exploring either the reason for the action or the due process system in place. But both employees were popular, and friends went to the media on their behalf. Taking a second look, I created an investigatory team to review both the original offenses and the discipline proposed; that report prompted a much lower level of discipline. The fact that I took a second look, that I met with the involved employees personally, and that I was open within the agency and with the media (within constraints of personnel law) were taken as positive signs. While this did not eliminate concern about the original action and my error in supporting it, it did establish a climate of openness to employee concerns and honesty about actions that were important to building staff constituency. Further, the media learned that I was accessible and began turning to the division for information and commentary on a more regular basis.

In the second case, just before a holiday weekend, I concurred in a staff recommendation to announce restrictions in use of drinking water in a coastal resort town. Several hotels and eating facilities were closed. While I did several of the "right" things, such as verifying the laboratory findings of fecal contamination of the water and alerting the department and governor's offices prior to any public announcement, there were problems. I did not know that this particular resort area was home to many "old Oregon" families, who expected to spend their Labor Day weekend as usual and did not appreciate my attempts to improve their health. I did not fully know the history of sanitary regulation in the county, where the Health Division had just assumed jurisdiction due to failure of the county health department to enforce regulations. This meant that in a small county, where people were used to familiar, face-to-face interactions, their first encounter with the new sanitarians was an announcement from Portland that their water was too dirty to use.

In hindsight, I should have ensured that personal calls were made to county commissioners and state legislators from the area (one of whom was on my budget committee); I should also have sought a negotiated interim plan for water management prior to the public warning. As it was, all planning for an upgraded water system and reopening of public eating facilities were conducted under media and legislative scrutiny. Strong voices argued that I was one more example of big city, big government run amok. Over a year later, I joined a number of state, federal, and local officials in dedicating the town's new water treatment plant, one of the best in the state. The long-term, constituency-building impact of this incident was to affirm to the public health community that I would support appropriate public health actions, and to the political community that I would honestly own the negative effects of my communication decisions—without backing down on protecting the public's health.

RELATIONSHIPS WITH LOCAL HEALTH DEPARTMENTS

Local health departments are important partners of state health agencies, tailoring programs to local needs and priorities that may vary widely across a state. In Oregon, local government is a very important constituency for all state agencies, and the Oregon Conference of Local Health Officials (CLHO) was an active member of the Association of Counties. As mentioned earlier, this group had become quite critical of the Health Division structure within the Department of Human Resources and was concerned that the division pay more attention to local needs and become a more vocal advocate for resources. In the legislative session just prior to my appointment, they had succeeded in creating a general subsidy for local public health (at the small sum of $0.25/capita/year), and they expected the Health Division to advocate for an increase in this fund.

A county commissioner and a local health director were on the interview panel that assisted in my hiring process, and it was made clear that I needed to develop a good relationship with staff throughout the state. For that reason, I set the goal of visiting each of the local health departments serving Oregon's 36 counties. These visits, which took a year to complete and limited my time with my own staff, provided an important firsthand view of the local health department partners in the state. In addition, I made a point of attending public health meetings within the state, including the annual CLHO meeting, held in conjunction with the state Public Health Association meeting. These interactions, which were a marked change from my predecessors, contributed to a common base of understanding of what might be done, or should be done, on behalf of public health in Oregon.

The shift in federal funding to block grants in the early 1980s led to one of the first tests of the relationship that was emerging. Before that time, federal funds for local public health were made available on a competitive basis. My travels had revealed the serious flaw in the method: Those departments that had a stronger infrastructure were able to compete and win more resources, and smaller departments scraped by on the minimum available. The look at statewide priorities necessitated by the conversion to block grants allowed us to consider the use of a formula approach, which could assure Oregonians equitable access to supported services regardless of which county they lived in. Appointment of an advisory committee with representation from local health departments of several sizes, as well as other interest groups, provided the forum for discussing and eventually designing a workable allocation system that could be phased in over several years.

The emerging statewide public health constituency supported a collaborative effort to ensure that no public health block grant funds would be diverted elsewhere and that the maximum possible amount of additional state funds would augment the amount to be distributed by the new formula. Had state funds been available, this would have also been the time to increase the general public health funding, but the statewide economic recession made this impossible.

The struggle over the balance between local public health and the state health division continued. While the local health departments wanted a strong voice for public health, they would have preferred that the voice only raise issues central to local concerns and advocate solely for local resources. Caught up in local struggles to support county allocations for public health, they often lost sight of the need for resources at the state level for activities with which they had little day-to-day contact. There were conflicting agendas among the local representatives, without a single voice from any one county being evident. For example, the administrator might agree with a priority-setting exercise for the budget, in which cutting back on support for dental health or swimming pool inspections made sense to preserve critical epidemiology, infectious disease control, and drinking-water consultation capacities. Yet in public testimony or meetings, other officials from that same administrator's agency might vehemently attack the state budget decisions as irrational and irresponsible. Statewide professional associations of nurses, sanitarians, or public health professionals were at times used as the vehicle for these contradictory messages.

The continuing confrontation led to an extraordinary meeting of the local health directors (without any other supervisory staff) and the executive staff of the Health Division. At this retreat, we reconfirmed our awareness of the damage we could do to public health by not forming a solid, mutually supportive constituency, what we called a "public health management team for the state." State and county officials chaired alternately, working on a mutually developed agenda. Items could only be added if they were of interest to more than one county or to more than one state program, and if there was evidence that an effort had been made to resolve the issue at a lower level. While these may sound like obvious ground rules, making them explicit gave the entire group a share in controlling maverick members who might care more about singling out an issue than developing a stronger public health system. This forum worked well to defuse arguments and push staff at both state and county levels to work collaboratively.

A PUBLIC HEALTH ADVISORY BOARD

Advocates for public health in Oregon often referred fondly to the "good old days," when a governor-appointed board of health had regulatory authority in public health and assisted in hiring and supervising the director. The board had been eliminated when the Health Division became a part of Department of Human Resources, in part because of management studies suggesting that the independent board or commission form of government previously popular in Oregon did not allow the governor to effectively manage the executive branch. What was lost was a public forum for debate of public health issues.

A board of health, even one lacking administrative power, can explore issues publicly, giving voice to alternatives and providing a place where those interested in public health issues can seek attention. Unlike legislative hearings, which are tied to the political agendas of the participants even under the best of circumstances, or regulatory hearings, which are tied to rules or specific cases, a board of health can explore issues in advance of any decision needed and can provide opportunities for education and information-sharing. It took a number of years of building relationships before the idea of reestablishing a board of health could be successfully broached, first within the executive branch and then later with the legislature.

Use of advisory committees has long been a part of public life in Oregon. The strong open meetings and sunshine laws meant that interested parties could follow or participate in matters being considered by public officials. The Health Division had established a tradition of using advisory bodies regularly, even when not required by law. My approach was to consider all meetings open unless there were a strong legal reason otherwise (such as having a personnel issue under consideration). Work done on revising the state's drinking water laws, developing a statewide trauma system, and revising local health funding formulas all included use of advisory committees representative of divergent interests. None of these bodies could develop a long-term, statewide, public health view, however. And while the CLHO clearly had long-term and statewide views, it was hard for them to step out of their local government positions to look at other issues. Establishment of a public health advisory board would provide a common forum for all of these and other interests and would reduce the need to establish shorter-term groups.

Once established by the legislature and appointed, the Public Health Advisory Board (PHAB) did begin to provide a wider voice for public health issues. Its members were in a position to take public health issues back to their constituencies, including the CLHO, individual professional associations, and the Association of Counties, educating them about the role of public health in the public life of the state.

LONG-TERM RESULTS

Two long-term results of constituency building are cited here: the development of state goals for Healthy People 2000 and Oregon's updated disease-reporting laws. Each accomplishment benefited from the constituency building activities reported above.

Oregon was the first state in the nation to publish health goals for the year 2000. These were developed in the late 1980s, during the time when the national Healthy People 2000 goals were under development. Oregon had not done anything specific to adapt the goals for 1990 to the state, mostly because there were higher priorities for action early in the decade, and as time went on it seemed less important to do so. Many in the state also felt that the format for the existing national goals was too bureaucratic to be useful. In 1988 I challenged a small group of Oregonians, including representatives from the state's PHAB and CLHO and advocates for several age groups (children, the elderly) to identify a relatively small number of goals that the state should try to achieve by the end of the century. The resultant publication, which was both eye-catching and readable, triggered a great deal of attention and provided a useful template for budget and organizational decisions. It also became an early part of the state's discussion of the statewide goal-setting process, in which Oregon is leading the nation. It is unlikely that the Health Division would have succeeded in publishing any widely read and used document if it had not developed the constituencies for public health in the preceding years.

In the early years of the human immunodeficiency virus (HIV) epidemic, many states struggled with questions about the appropriateness of applying old communicable disease control statutes to current realities. Oregon was one of those states. There had been some interest in updating laws to include noncommunicable diseases and conditions such as chemical exposures, injury, and birth defects. Advocates for those with HIV infection wanted to be assured that no arbitrary reporting or limitation of liberty would be imposed on those at risk of HIV. Use of a widely based working group, which included those with HIV infection and their caregivers, members of professional associations, members of bar and civil liberties associations, and others, provided a forum for debating possible statutory adjustments. In the end, a bill was sent to the legislature that proposed completely rewriting statutes covering "conditions of public health importance."

The new law ensured that any reporting was confidential and that any imposition of restrictions on an individual with a communicable condition was done only after all voluntary efforts failed and in the least restrictive manner possible. The law allowed for flexibility in specific regulations over time, rather than spelling out all details in the law. In front of the key legislative committee, representatives of many constituencies (some in almost constant conflict with one another in other settings) concurred that this statute was appropriate and should be passed; it was. The Oregon law is now mentioned by analysts of HIV legislation as one of the best in the nation. Without the support of a public health constituency to say that HIV must be considered in conjunction with other public health issues, and without the constituency support to take time to work through issues prior to legislative consideration, it is unlikely that this law would ever have been passed. Oregon might well have been saddled with some of the problematic reporting or restriction laws passed elsewhere.

LESSONS LEARNED

The level of funding available for public health through the budget-cutting years; the strong laws on conditions of public health importance, on trauma systems, and on drinking water protection; and the enthusiastic involvement of Oregon public health practitioners in national efforts to improve public health all speak to the strengthening of constituencies for public health in the state. Further evidence comes from the involvement of public health officials in devising the Oregon plan for extension of medical care benefits to the poor and in planning for revisions of Medicaid funding. In Oregon's benchmarking approach to statewide goal achievement, public health activities are seen as essential to achieving goals: Given the state's interest in assuring that all children are prepared to learn in school, and to stay in school, support for child health and adolescent pregnancy prevention programs has been very strong.

The role played by any one individual in building public health over a decade is relatively small; many dedicated individuals committed themselves to the effort.

There are, however, some things that were probably best done by or with the direct support of the agency director. I learned how difficult it is to keep an eye on the overall goal and work toward a long-term result. For example, as the interest in public health grew in the state, many local environmental health workers wanted to move quickly to rewrite the state's very weak drinking water protection law. I wanted that law rewritten, and I wanted the support of local environmental health workers. However, my assessment was that this effort would not be successful until a better track record under the existing program was in place, and after some of the year-to-year budget consistency discussed above had been demonstrated. With great effort, it was possible to hold back the enthusiasts while developing the legislative package that eventually passed. Had the question been raised before my encounter with residents and legislators over the quality of the coastal water system, I believe my enthusiasm would have led me to join local lobbying efforts, and we would have needlessly lost an important struggle.

Another important lesson is that of mastering multiple vocabularies and communication styles. Many of us are familiar with profiling used to identify the various preferred work and communication styles of people who find themselves working together. It took me a long time to understand fully the enormous gap that can occur when these differences are not taken into account. Many public health practitioners are trained in scientific disciplines, in which details and factual evidence predominate. Work in the decision-making arena of government involves a large number of people for whom intuition is more important than evidence. Constituency building means crossing those lines and finding ways for the detail-oriented individuals to feel comfortable without driving the big-picture enthusiasts crazy with repetition. My interest in getting on with things often frustrated epidemiologists and others who wanted to be sure I understood all the details; I was often too willing to assume that something said once had been understood and agreed to by those in the room. Learning mutual ground rules within the public health community strengthened our ability to work with the outside constituency when we needed to make desired improvements.

Constituencies are built around clear goals and need positive feedback and flexible support over time. As state health director, I had extraordinary opportunities to support the emergence of a constituency for public health. This case report has described some of the activities and opportunities I was able to use to strengthen public health in Oregon. It could only be done by making myself visible and vulnerable to criticism, open to change and input, and willing to collaborate creatively, even with those holding strongly differing opinions. It was an experience well worth the effort.

PART II

Confronting Crisis

Confronting Crisis

CHAPTER 4

Confronting a Border Health Crisis: A Comprehensive Approach

Jack Dillenberg and Douglas Hirano

In October 1993, the border community of Nogales, Arizona, began receiving national notoriety as a community with unexplained, unusually high numbers of residents with diseases such as systemic lupus erythematosus (SLE), multiple myeloma, and leukemia. News accounts appeared in *USA Today* and on the Discovery Channel, as well as in regional newspapers. In these stories, residents pointed to sewage-contaminated river washes, burning landfills, and pollution-producing *maquiladoras* (American-owned factories along the Mexican border) as possible reasons for the high disease rates. Preliminary data gathered by the University of Arizona seemed to bear out that the lupus rates were elevated; indeed, the rates were being quoted as the highest in the world.

In December 1993, Arizona Governor Fife Symington, Senator John McCain, and key staff from the Arizona Department of Health Services (ADHS) and the Arizona Department of Environmental Quality (ADEQ) toured Nogales and met with residents, who spoke of entire neighborhoods plagued by a rare cancer known as multiple myeloma. Jimmy Teyechea, a local resident dying of multiple myeloma, pointed out houses with cancer victims in his Carrillo Street neighborhood. Moved by the depth and the scope of the Nogales community's problems, Governor Symington pledged $100,000 to conduct a thorough study of the disease problems and promised full funding of the ADHS cancer registry. In addition, he and Manlio Fabio Beltrones, the governor of Sonora, Mexico, created the Governors' Bi-national Task Force on Border Health to monitor progress and make recommendations regarding health between Sonora and Arizona.

Upon returning from this visit, two things had become clear: The ADHS would be making Nogales a priority issue over the next several months and, given the human, scientific, and political urgencies and complexities of the situation, the skills of a relatively new health director would be tested.

OVERVIEW

It is the rare state health department that will not eventually become embroiled in a cancer cluster investigation. I use the term "embroiled" because cancer cluster investigations are typically both politically and scientifically demanding. The elements of such an investigation often include community claims of unusual and excessive disease occurrences, suspicions that the disease is linked to industrial pollution, and, finally, claims of government inaction and cover-up. The media frequently depict government response as sluggish and unsympathetic to the plight of the public.

Now, if such investigations frequently resulted in an elucidated disease cause and risk-reducing interventions, then full-fledged investigation would be demanded. Unfortunately, few investigations can determine why a disease is occurring at a high rate. Even when a disease excess is confirmed, a specific disease etiology is rarely identified. Thus, the well-meaning concerns of residents are rarely satisfied, nor is disease risk decreased, yet significant time and resources end up being devoted to the investigation. This is a classic "no win" situation.

Consequently, in this situation, we realized that success could not be measured solely in terms of clean science, epidemiology, and disease prevention. Other important criteria included the development of a credible and trusting relationship with the Nogales community, the media, and the Sonoran health department; the procurement of federal health agency assistance and resources; and, ideally, development of a model for future border health work.

THE NOGALES COMMUNITY

Nogales, Arizona, is a border town in Santa Cruz County with a population of 19,489. According to the 1990 census, 92 percent of the inhabitants are Hispanic and 7.2 percent white, non-Hispanic. Nogales, Arizona, is adjacent to Nogales, Sonora, Mexico, which is a rapidly growing city; the official census population there is 107,000, but informal estimates are as high as 200,000. This rapid growth is attributed to the migration of people from southern Mexico who perceive Sonora as offering economic opportunity. The unfortunate outcome is that the burgeoning population is outstripping the city's infrastructure, particularly its sewage systems.

At any given time, the population numbers of both towns fluctuate greatly, since the border is fluid and thousands move across the border daily for work or to shop. There are more than 60 twin plants located in Nogales, Sonora, that employ over 20,000 people from both sides of the border. Nogales is also the major port of entry for produce imports along the international border; the fruits and vegetables that pass through Nogales are distributed throughout the United States. At the height of the winter season, approximately 800 trucks pass through Nogales each day. It is of particular significance that Nogales, Arizona, is downwind and downriver from Nogales, Sonora.

As already stated, by late 1993, the Nogales, Arizona, community was in pain: Neighbors, relatives, and friends were chronically ill or dying of rare diseases. Coupled with longstanding concerns about environmental pollution (e.g., burning landfills, truck exhaust at the border inspection station, sewage in the wash flowing northward from Mexico, and industrial pollution from the *maquiladoras*), residents assumed long-term exposure to the polluted environment was finally causing excess disease. People's powerlessness in the face of having to breathe unhealthy air, drink unsafe water, and eat potentially unclean food further created anger and resentment. Bad feeling was directed both at Mexico, for its lack of regulation of the *maquiladoras* and for its burning landfills and flowing sewage, and at the Arizona government, for its inability to move rapidly to address these problems.

It became clear that the department was sitting on a powder keg. Jimmy Teyechea, the self-designated community spokesman, was getting sicker, and his deteriorating health magnified the urgency and seriousness of the situation. He had already been lionized by the local and national media, and he had begun attacking ADHS epidemiologists in angry letters to the governor's office. At the same time, however, rumblings from the Nogales business community were occurring, criticizing the advocacy community for characterizing Nogales as a "cancer town" in the national press. The expanding retail and tourist business in Nogales was at risk if Nogales developed a reputation as an unhealthy and possibly dangerous business and tourist location.

Given the danger of negative public opinion, I realized that the proper ADHS role would be to conduct a scientifically rigorous disease study and to communicate the results to the public and the media in understandable terms. This would be our best bet to avoid exaggerated characterizations of the disease problem in Nogales, which could further polarize the situation. Of course, ADHS was not the only agency with an interest in and a responsibility for addressing the Nogales situation. Many other agencies were actively involved in the Nogales health problem.

THE UNIVERSITY OF ARIZONA

The University of Arizona, particularly its rural health office and cancer center, had been active in Nogales for many years, working closely with the community in leading community-based health initiatives and research. In many ways, Nogales, which is only a one-hour drive from Tucson, served as an informal and convenient "laboratory" for the university to conduct rural and border health programs and research. As early as 1988, university researchers had been investigating possible cancer clusters in Nogales. In 1988, investigative activities were conducted to examine rates of pancreatic cancer; however, after formal case confirmation activities were completed, they were unable to verify a statistically significant increase in disease rates.

In early 1993, the university's Cancer Center had contacted the ADHS Office of Chronic Disease Epidemiology, stating their suspicion that excessive cancer rates were occurring in Nogales. However, a comparison of county-specific cancer mortality rates did not indicate excessive overall cancer mortality in the Nogales area, nor did a county-specific comparison of anencephaly rates uncover any unusual disease rates in Nogales. Clearly, however, the University of Arizona had great interest in disease patterns in Nogales and felt responsible for the health of the community. As we would see, the university was well known in Nogales for its community-based approach to research and programs. This community rapport would have important implications concerning the conduct of the disease study.

THE ARIZONA DEPARTMENT OF ENVIRONMENTAL QUALITY

Fortuitously, the ADEQ was already developing a comprehensive program in Nogales to sample air, water, and soil. Their efforts were supported in large part by funding from the U.S. Environmental Protection Agency. In fact, air sampling was to be conducted on both sides of the border. Water sampling already had begun in order to document the extent of trichloroethylene contamination of the water table on the Arizona side of the border. Consequently, we were hopeful that the combination of this environmental data and our disease study data would strengthen the likelihood of finding environmental links to the alleged increased disease rates.

In addition, ADEQ had been strengthening its relations with border communities. The department was conducting environmental "open houses," giving the public an opportunity to discuss environmental information in an informal setting with scientists. This type of forum was proving useful in gaining community trust. The department was also planning on stationing staff in Nogales to coordinate sampling activities. This included the development of a border office to house local environmental data and staff. The ADHS would later agree to co-fund the office.

And finally, it was helpful that Ed Fox, then director of the ADEQ, had a close working relationship with ADHS staff. Fox is a respected and trusted figure in Arizona environmental issues. We both agreed that the Nogales situation required tender, loving care, and I felt sure that his thoughts and recommendations regarding this situation would be critically important to our overall success.

SECRETARÍA DE SALUD PÚBLICA DE SONORA

The Sonorans were clearly in a difficult position. Many Nogales residents blamed pollution from Mexico as the cause of the high disease rates. However, as already stated, lack of resources for sanitation systems, water treatment, and a new landfill hampered Sonora's ability to effect the changes that they wanted. After all, the lack of proper sanitation, alleged groundwater contamination, and burning landfills would theoretically affect Nogales, Sonora, residents as well as Nogales, Arizona, residents.

The Sonoran health department officials were caught in the middle. They supported new resources for environmental and infrastructure improvements, but they also depended on Mexico's federal officials to approve funds for these projects. Tragically, Luis Colosio, a leading presidential candidate from Sonora, was assassinated in March 1994. Local Sonorans believed his successful candidacy would have brought heightened federal attention to the pressing needs of the city.

Thankfully, staff from the Secretaría de Salud Pública (SSP) were most cooperative in investigating the possible disease problem. They rapidly conducted a preliminary review of cancer and lupus cases on the Sonora side, which did not indicate statistically significant disease excesses.

As a footnote, it should be mentioned that the collaboration between ADHS and SSP was exemplary and eventually extended beyond the Nogales situation. We have since worked jointly on numerous other disease problems, and Dr. Ernesto Rivera-Claisse, the Sonoran health director, has become a special ally to the department. This was one of the unexpected benefits of taking a bi-national approach to the problem.

THE SANTA CRUZ COUNTY HEALTH DEPARTMENT

Like many small county health departments, the Santa Cruz County Health Department did not have full-time staff available to conduct complex investigations of disease clusters. Therefore, the county health department, which is located in Nogales, was not in a position to provide significant assistance in the disease study. However, the county health director served an important role by reminding the local media of the potential health problems related to long-term exposure to burning landfills, polluted river washes, and bad air. To the extent possible, therefore, the county health director was assisting community efforts by serving as a strong advocate for environmental clean-up. This advocacy role occasionally meant calling on state and federal agencies to clean up the environment and to provide political impetus for Mexico to do the same. This occasionally created frustration since we at ADHS and those at ADEQ felt we were doing all we could to deal with the many issues swirling around the disease problems in Nogales. To the credit of all involved, local, state, and federal agencies generally worked well together and kept a balanced perspective about the broader goals of disease investigation, environmental assessment, and caring for the sick.

THE LIFE GROUP

The LIFE (Living Is For Everyone) group arose directly from community concerns about the environment and disease excesses. Jimmy Teyechea and Anna Acuña, a lupus sufferer, spearheaded the organization of the group, with Acuña becoming the executive director in light of Teyechea's deteriorating health and eventual death in March 1994.

LIFE served as the community conscience in regard to the disease and how concerns about its prevalence were being addressed. However, the LIFE group was relatively small and new; moreover, it was essentially run on a shoestring budget. Its efforts were initially focused on serving as an informational resource for persons suffering from multiple myeloma and lupus. Acuña attended meetings and advocated for medical resources for the care and treatment of disease sufferers, for elucidation of the cause of disease, and for environmental clean-up.

Although LIFE was a relatively small organization, we knew that we would have to keep its members informed of the higher disease rates throughout our investigation. They could make or break our relationship with the broader community and adversely affect participation in the planned disease study.

DEVELOPMENT OF THE DISEASE STUDY

With regard to the disease study ordered by Governor Symington, our epidemiologists first recommended confirmation of increased rates of disease and then suggested a case/control study to identify potential risk factors for such an increase. To remain within the prescribed time limitation suggested by the governor, who wanted a full report by the end of June 1994, we realized we had to move quickly. Since the University of Arizona Cancer Center had already conducted a preliminary assessment of lupus incidence in Nogales and had established a relationship with the community, it seemed logical to utilize the center to conduct the disease confirmation and case/control study.

The Cancer Center was in fact quite willing to conduct the study but had a different idea about how to approach it. They did not believe that a case/control study, with the small numbers involved, would yield statistically significant results. Therefore, they suggested a study protocol, whose structure would be more research oriented. This community survey protocol included the drawing of blood from study subjects in Nogales and in Patagonia, a comparison community, in order to test for biochemical markers for preclinical lupus, for future onset of multiple myeloma, and for geographic correlation of those with biochemical markers with "community-defined areas of environmental concern." While we believed this to be an interesting approach, we felt strongly that our public health obligation ought to rapidly conduct a case/control study to identify potentially preventable risk factors. The university, perhaps believing the money to be available only through one-time funding, wanted to pursue the larger study.

After several weeks of negotiation, some of it quite stressful, a compromise was reached. The case/control study, including in-depth subject interviews, would be "nested" in the larger study, which included blood draws for biochemical markers and community assessments of areas of environmental concern. Unfortunately, the Nogales media found out about the rift in study approaches and criticized both agencies for "butting heads" while the public wanted and needed answers. This would not be the last time we suffered negative press.

The university's case follow-up investigation eventually confirmed statistically significant excesses of lupus and multiple myeloma occurring in the Nogales, Arizona, area. The increased rates of lupus largely took place among Hispanic women, which was somewhat difficult to place in perspective, since race-specific rates of lupus were not available in the literature. However, the stage was now set for the community study, which would include a case/control investigation as well as biochemical marker testing.

THE ADHS COMMUNITY STRATEGY

As previously stated, the perceived increase in disease and its alleged ties to environmental ills brought with it numerous other issues: tourist industry concerns about Nogales being viewed as a "cancer" town, the smoldering anger of long-time residents who believed any response would be "too little too late," the lack of health care for the uninsured and undocumented, the limited resources available through the local health department, and the binational politics of enforcing environmental standards in Mexico and developing new sewage plants and landfills on the Mexican side of the border.

Consequently, I had to decide whether we would take a minimalist approach, focusing primarily on the completion of the disease study, or take a more comprehensive approach. As stated earlier, investigations of cancer or other chronic disease clusters are often labor intensive and rarely provide the satisfaction of identifying and preventing disease. This predisposed us toward taking a minimalist approach. However, the high-profile, political nature of the matter suggested otherwise. An excess of neural tube defects in the Matamoros/Brownsville area of Texas had already heightened federal interest in investigating potential environmentally provoked disease along the border. In addition, Governor Symington had an expressed interest in developing strong relations with the Sonorans, particularly in the economic arena, and Nogales was the major gateway between Sonora and Arizona. The merits of the proposed North American Free Trade Agreement (NAFTA) were being hotly debated, and the controversy suggested that health along the border would be a continuing concern. It appeared that our efforts in Nogales needed to be comprehensive; we also felt that we could serve as a model for public health efforts in other border health localities. However, we realized that we could not solve all the ills of the community. We had to combine the provision of scientific and technical assistance in the conduct of a rigorous disease investigation with a compassionate good faith effort to deal with other related community concerns.

Our first step was to get our own house at ADHS in order. We formed an internal health services working group on Nogales, which included public information and community relations staff, environmental health specialists, local health liaisons, health promotion specialists, our state epidemiologist, and staff from the director's office. This multidisciplinary group, which met regularly over the next year and a half, planned community and binational meetings, coordinated the disease study with the University of Arizona, dealt with the community and the media, and communicated with local and Sonoran health officials. We included representatives from the ADEQ and the Arizona Radiation Regulatory Agency at planning meetings to make sure we were coordinating efforts.

Initially, the group decided that the ADHS needed to deal immediately with the underlying pain and hardship within the community. With that in mind, key staff traveled to Nogales to meet with community leaders to discuss community needs relating to the disease cluster. The community leaders decided that medical assistance was needed, and we provided funds for University of Arizona staff to offer rheumatological and oncological consultation to patients with lupus and cancer in Nogales. (University personnel traveled to Nogales once a week for this purpose.) This consultation fulfilled the community's perceived need for care and also maintained the community's connection with the University of Arizona. It also sent the message that the ADHS was willing to pitch in to assist the community, regardless of the eventual outcome of the study. The ADHS director personally participated in all activities, particularly meetings with the community in Nogales. We felt it was important that the director of the ADHS be highly visible throughout our response to the problems.

In addition to medical consultation, the community also requested assistance in educating people regarding environmental health issues and in assisting persons with lupus and cancer in identifying resources for psychological and social support. Consequently, we contracted with the LIFE group to provide these services. This contract supported the fledgling organization and also provided the community with needed services.

To expand the effort of establishing a working relationship with the Nogales community, the ADHS and the ADEQ collaborated with the Secretaría de Salud Pública de Sonora to hold two open houses—one in Nogales, Arizona, and one in Nogales, Sonora. These open houses were meant to provide an informal outlet for community members to talk about important issues with health department and agency staff monitoring environmental quality from both sides of the border. We also arranged for staff from our Medicaid agency to be on hand to field any questions regarding eligibility for Medicaid services. Public information staff from all agencies involved made sure that all printed materials were bilingual and culturally appropriate. Attendance at the Nogales, Arizona, open house was good. Interestingly, the Sonorans took a more festive approach and held a more traditional health fair on the Sonoran side of the border. This drew more people, including children, and created a fun atmosphere—an interesting counterpoint to our more low-key approach.

Last, to create a more stable presence in Nogales, the ADEQ and the ADHS leased a trailer in downtown Nogales, where the community could find environmental information available. This trailer also served as an office for visiting ADEQ and ADHS staff. Ultimately, the office served as a symbol of the joint and ongoing commitment of the ADEQ and the ADHS to resolve the health problems in Nogales. In general, the attempts to address community concerns (above and beyond the disease study) were well received and seemed to enhance our credibility. These initiatives also served to solidify our relationship with the ADEQ and the Sonoran health department staff. This set the stage for the completion of the disease study and the dissemination of the results.

STUDY RESULTS AND DISSEMINATION

In December 1994, the final report was completed by the University of Arizona. This was six months after the date Governor Symington requested, but realistically was quite expedient given the ambitiousness of the study.

Statistically significant increases in the number of lupus and multiple myeloma cases in the Nogales area were confirmed by the University of Arizona. The biochemical testing of study subjects suggested statistically significant numbers of Nogales women with elevated titers of antinuclear antibody (ANA), a subclinical marker for lupus, as compared to women living in Patagonia, the nearby control community. The residence of women with elevated ANA titers was geographically associated with community-defined areas of environmental concern and with existing lupus cases. University researchers concluded that adverse health effects had in fact occurred in Nogales and that they resulted from complex environmental exposures to biological or chemical agents. However, no specific etiology was identified. Further, while comprehensive questionnaires were administered to subjects from Nogales and

Patagonia, no data analyses were conducted concerning occupational, environmental, family history, or other potential risk factors.

Concerning the study, we felt that we had accomplished much in a short period of time; however, we were fearful that the community would demand that the cause of the higher disease rates be found. We had no answers, and ultimately we believed *how* we presented the information would be as important as *what* we presented. Consequently, we decided that the community should be the first to hear the results of our study. This turned out to be a bit difficult, as the local media demanded the results a day before the planned community meeting in order to meet publishing deadlines. We felt it was critically important that the very first news of our findings be reported directly to the community, and so we decided not to make our information public until the community meeting.

At the meeting, the University of Arizona researchers took the lead in explaining the study results, but only brought about 20 copies to the community forum. Yet many among the approximately 80 media and community members present wanted their own copy. While we realized that the report was written for the scientific reader, we felt strongly that copies should be available to all. The director loaned a credit card to a university staff member to make additional copies at a local copy shop. This gesture was appreciated and quieted the grumblings of the audience. In the end, the public seemed satisfied that we had confirmed a true increase in disease rates. The audience also seemed pleased that the ADHS was going to take these study findings to the federal government, in the hope of getting funds to study the disease and to assist with medical care for the sick and dying. Little attention was given to the fact that we had not yet isolated the cause of disease. However, the public in Nogales also wanted time to study the report and have an opportunity to discuss it again. We promised that we would be back within 100 days to discuss the matter more thoroughly.

The ADHS director was scheduled to attend a conference at the Centers for Disease Control and Prevention (CDC) in Atlanta the very next day, and he told the audience that he was bringing copies of the report to Atlanta, where he would hand deliver them to Dr. David Satcher, the CDC director; to Dr. Phil Lee, the Assistant Secretary for the Department of Health and Human Services (DHHS); and to Dr. Richard Jackson, the head of the CDC's Center for Environmental Health. When he saw each of these individuals the next day, he gave them a simple message: "Texas is not the only state with border health problems." He decided on a simple but pointed quote because it was not clear that their busy schedules would have permitted an immediate and thorough review of the document.

One hundred days later, in March 1995, we returned to Nogales to further discuss the study with community members. Along with us was the CDC epidemiologist, Dr. Rossanne Philen, who substantiated the report's usefulness in confirming disease problems and supported our request for greater attention from federal agencies. Philen, who speaks fluent Spanish, answered a community member's question in that language. This won over the audience and paved the way for a successful meeting. Toward the end of the meeting, he promised the community that the ADHS would recruit a CDC Epidemic Intelligence Service (EIS) Officer to work on further research needs in Nogales.

EPILOGUE

Much has happened since the release of the study report, and almost all of it is positive. While we ultimately were unable to recruit an EIS officer, we did hire an exceptional bilingual medical epidemiologist. His job is to study border epidemiology issues, with an immediate focus on Nogales. In addition, the CDC agreed to pay half of his salary. In cooperation with the Sonoran health department, a border epidemiological research office has recently been established in Sonora—the first of its kind along the border between the United States and Mexico. We believe all this resulted directly from the hand delivery of the report to top U.S. Public Health Service officials, as well as from letters and phone calls requesting assistance in the study's follow-up. Again, the overriding message we attempted to deliver to federal officials was that Texas is not the only state with border health issues.

This message and associated advocacy efforts also led to a meeting in Tucson of the Interagency Coordinating Committee on environmental health along the border. This was the first time this group had ever met in Arizona. Key members of the group, which included officials from the Environmental Protection Agency (EPA), the CDC, and other federal agencies, agreed to stay an extra day to tour Nogales and meet with community members there.

We have also continued to support the care and treatment of lupus sufferers in Nogales through a contract with the community health center there. With funding from the Agency for Toxic Substances and Disease Registry (ATSDR), we've maintained efforts to educate the general public and health professionals about environmental issues. With approval from the ATSDR, an ADHS community environmental health specialist splits her time between Nogales and Tucson to build local capacity to address environmental issues. We've also since established the ADHS Border Health Office. Our presence in the area is strong and stable.

SUMMARY

While this sounds like a happy ending to a difficult scenario, we must be honest and state that our response in Nogales came at some cost. Certainly, the director's time and the time of key staffers could have been productively spent on other matters. The likelihood of actual delineation of the disease's cause and its prevention was quite small from the beginning. Clearly, environmental clean-up needed to happen in the Nogales area regardless of the results of the disease study. In fact, additional resources along the border for environmental clean-up and infrastructure development still await funding, but that matter is in the hands of federal officials.

That being said, we firmly believe the benefits from the overall disease study were well worth the time and effort. We have established enhanced relations with ADEQ, the Secretaría de Salud Pública de Sonora, the Nogales community, the CDC Center for Environmental Health, and the University of Arizona. Additionally, we have new internal resources to extend the disease study and enhance border health activities generally, and the Nogales community has a greater capacity to deal with environmental health issues.

Ultimately, our response is a model for treating a suspected environmental disease cluster as a community health crisis. The broad-based approach successfully united the Nogales community, Sonoran health officials, state agencies such as the ADHS and the ADEQ, and the University of Arizona in confronting an issue of great community concern.

CHAPTER 5

Crisis of Confidence: Neural Tube Defects in South Texas

David R. Smith

In April 1991, a Texas physician and a nurse in Brownsville (Cameron County) alerted the Texas Department of Health (TDH) about an apparent cluster of fatal birth defects. The physician had witnessed the birth of three anencephalic infants within 36 hours. Anencephaly is one of two common neural tube defects (NTDs), which are birth defects of the brain and/or spinal cord that frequently lead to death or disability; the other is spina bifida. NTDs are major contributors to state and national infant mortality statistics.

This incident and similar reports from Brownsville within a six-week period sparked a history-making campaign by the TDH to identify the causes of NTDs and develop interventions to address the high incidence of these birth defects in Cameron County. The location magnified the severity of the reports. Located in the southernmost area of Texas, Cameron County shares its border with Mexico. Most of the population (84.5 percent) is Mexican-American, and half of the adults over 25 years of age have not completed high school. The area is known for its high poverty rate; the median income is less than $11,000. Thousands live in *colonias*—unincorporated areas characterized by substandard housing, roads, drainage, and water and sewer systems—and are exposed to unsafe and unsanitary environmental conditions. Cameron County experiences higher rates of illness and disease than do other areas of the state. In several areas of the county the number of health care professionals is inadequate.

The people of Cameron and surrounding counties have many unmet health care needs and have long suffered from neglect. The general perception in this region is that government and academic officials spend more time studying and characterizing problems than solving them. Over time, many citizens have come to believe that government does not care about them or their health.

When I first learned of the NTD crisis in Cameron County, I sensed that the issue was larger than the simple identification of its cause. The critical issue was one of confidence and trust. Given the current perceptions of government and its ability to effect change in the Lower Rio Grande Valley, I understood the skepticism felt by local residents. Yet I also recognized a cry for help. Our agency could use this crisis to bring needed attention and resources to the area, or we could find ourselves in the middle of a major political struggle.

Some residents had predetermined that toxins emitted by *maquiladoras* (Mexican factories, often American owned) caused the high incidence of NTDs. These activists feared that officials would protect the interests of the chemical and manufacturing plants, not those of the citizens. They had begun to mobilize against these factories, putting themselves at odds with some local politicians, business people, and professional colleagues. Attorneys were gravitating to both sides of the issue. This struggle occurred at a time of heated debate over the North American Free Trade Agreement (NAFTA), which further heightened emotions and conflict between public and private interests.

The headlines magnified and distorted reality as major networks and nationally syndicated news columns published a story about the crisis entitled "Babies Born without Brains." I knew that this volatile situation required immediate attention. I was angered by the failure of many reporters to distinguish between truth and popular perception. Contrary to the information in many published articles, the actual increase in cases of anencephaly occurred miles to the north of Brownsville, in northern Cameron County.

My interest in the NTD campaign was both personal and professional. This was not a remote community I had never heard of and would never visit; Cameron County was once my home. My wife and I had practiced in the Lower Rio Grande Valley for more than three years. I had become an active member of the community and had served on the school board. Many people knew me on a first-name basis and had come to trust and respect me. I could not ignore their pleas for help. My personal reputation was on the line.

This campaign also represented one of the first major challenges confronting me as the newly appointed commissioner for the TDH. Many people in the state would be assessing my leadership abilities by looking at my decisions and actions in this crisis. I wanted to show that I could make a difference in a way that supported rather than violated our scientific process.

I was concerned about politics—the local political environment as well as political realities at the state level. Governor Ann Richards called me to make sure that I was personally involved in addressing the problem. The governor's office shared my concern that our colleagues in Washington might not react quickly enough. We were aware that all eyes would be on Austin to see how responsive state government would be to the pleas of our poorer constituents. My decision seemed simple: I could not ignore this problem. Delegating my authority was never an option, as I had decided early in my tenure as commissioner that I was not looking for a job into which I wanted to retire.

THE STAKES

During the early part of the NTD campaign, my role was best defined as that of "problem-solver and worrier." I spent the initial days of the campaign playing out various scenarios and thinking through what I believed were the major issues. I realized that there were many stakeholders interested in the outcome of our campaign. The core group included parents of babies with NTDs, as well as all expecting parents. We did not know the extent of NTDs in Cameron County, nor did we know the causes or epidemiology of the birth defects, so any couple expecting a child had heightened concerns about the health of their unborn infant. Our ignorance about this defect was frustrating.

Medical and health care providers in the valley were also stakeholders. They were anxious to solve the NTD puzzle. Local activists, business people, and investors had an interest in the outcome of our investigation. Since the NTD crisis was occurring in the midst of the NAFTA debates, these groups would be affected by our findings, especially if they indicated environmental causes. The scientific community was invested in the results of our campaign, as it would be an opportunity to generate new knowledge in the area of birth defects. Scientists at the TDH had an additional concern. They were waiting to see if I would support them by placing our scientific resolve above politics. Of course, state and federal agencies were major stakeholders, since we had the primary responsibility for solving the mystery of the apparently high incidence of anencephaly.

In addition to the many stakeholders, the campaign involved risks. As previous scientific studies have failed to define a cause for NTDs, there was a good chance that we would not find a single, simple cause for their occurrence in Cameron County. Most authorities believe that NTDs are multifactorial in origin, involving genetic and environmental precursors. There would probably be no "smoking gun." We knew we would have to define success differently. And we did. We decided that success would mean bringing attention to the health problems in the area, doing a better job of expanded surveillance, and establishing an ongoing presence in the valley to monitor health status.

STRATEGIES

From the beginning, I believed that communications would be key to any strategy we employed. We would need to share information with citizens and gain their input. Communication and coordination among state and federal agencies would be critical to ensure that agencies were not pitted against one another. I realized that the department would need to act quickly to regain the trust of the citizens. Only after we had begun to establish confidence among residents could we focus our attention on the other major objectives of identifying the causes of NTDs and improving the county's general health and environmental conditions. I traveled to the lower Rio Grande Valley so that people could have personal contact with the department through me. We scheduled press conferences and reports in the community affected by the crisis, rather than in Austin.

We established a task force of experts and scientists from the TDH, federal agencies, and other state agencies; we also included individuals from the border. At our first meeting in Dallas, we outlined the major issues and developed a plan of action. The task force was especially concerned about avoiding duplication of effort, addressing community needs, and eliminating misinformation.

The TDH initiated a two-prong approach to the NTD effort: One aspect focused on science, the other on communications. Our initial scientific effort, an investigation of the apparent cluster of fatal defects, resulted in our obtaining accurate information about the incidence of these defects in the area. The Centers for Disease Control and Prevention (CDC) and local health authorities helped with the investigation, which began in May 1991. The study had four components:

1. Surveillance (case finding) to define the magnitude of the problem in Cameron County, including a retrospective review of births back to 1986.
2. A case-control study to define parental risk factors.
3. A laboratory component to screen for nutritional and environmental factors.
4. An environmental component to evaluate data on air quality, possible soil contamination, water quality, pesticides, and aflatoxins.

We recognized the need to gather information from both sides of the border. Representatives from the TDH, staff from the medical branch of the University of Texas, and Mexican officials started meeting in 1992 to discuss joint surveillance of NTDs along the entire Texas-Mexico border. They agreed to share vital information and to reconvene to further define the surveillance system.

In July 1992, the TDH released the findings from the investigation. The epidemiology division estimated the rate of NTD incidence in Cameron County for 1986 through 1991 at about 19 per 10,000 live births; for 1990–1991, the rate was 27.1 per 10,000 births. Fears of a sudden epidemic proved false. However, the study did confirm a long-term high incidence of NTDs in the area (see Figure 5–1). Rates were two-and-a-half times the 1990–1991 national rates of approximately 8.0 per 10,000 births. The results of the initial investigation clearly indicated the need for further study. To better understand the epidemiology of NTDs, we expanded our inquiry to include neighboring Hidalgo County and increased the review of hospital records to cover a 10-year period.

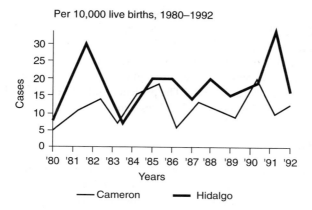

Figure 5–1 Prevalence Rates of NTD.

Since many residents believed pollution was the culprit responsible for increased incidence of NTDs, environmental assessment and monitoring studies were critical. The Texas Air Control Board and the Texas Water Commission (now combined as the Texas Natural Resources Conservation Commission) and the Texas Department of Agriculture cooperated by supplying environmental sampling data. The U.S. Environmental Protection Agency approved a water-quality study in the Rio Grande basin. We hoped that federal involvement would boost efforts to curb the ever-worsening health environment on the border. If nothing else, we wanted to reassure the citizens of Cameron County by placing a high priority on the environmental investigation.

Although the data did not support environmental causes for NTDs, the report did recommend environmental monitoring studies to characterize the potential impact of toxic industrial air emissions, particularly those from industry in the Brownsville-Matamoros area. Many local residents were disappointed that no clear environmental link to NTDs had been found, and the department was criticized as a result. Because so many residents were convinced that environmental pollution from factories caused the NTDs, no amount of data saying otherwise could sway their beliefs, and in spite of our report, in 1993 a number of families filed a multimillion dollar class action lawsuit against several companies with border plants, blaming them for the birth defects. In part, this suit stemmed from information released by some members of the academic community. Unfortunately, in at least two instances, academic researchers provided preliminary and incomplete data to the press, further complicating our investigative efforts and falsely biasing the public.

In response to one of the report's recommendations, I advocated the formation of an independent 11-member National Scientific Advisory Committee of experts to provide guidance for NTD surveillance and intervention projects. Two members of this committee, a physician and a priest, were from the Lower Rio Grande Valley. The advisory committee met three times during the campaign, holding one of its meetings in Cameron County. The presence and interest of this high-ranking group improved relations between local residents and governmental agencies.

THE PROGRAM

In 1991 the results of a large, prospective study were published in the *Lancet,* demonstrating that folic acid, a B vitamin, can reduce the risk of recurrence of NTDs when taken periconceptionally. Although the results of a Hungarian prospective trial showing that folic acid can also reduce the risk of first occurrence of NTDs were not published until December 1992, we had advance notice of this finding. The results of these two studies, combined with those of a number of earlier suggestive U.S. and international reports, led us to conclude that approximately 40 to 70 percent of the occurrences of NTDs could be prevented. To effectively reduce risk, we determined that women should consume 0.4 milligrams of folic acid every day from at least 30 days before conception through the first month of pregnancy, the time critical for neural tube development.

Initially, we believed we had found a way to make an immediate difference in our fight against NTDs. However, our jubilation subsided as both border residents and some members of the scientific community began to criticize us. Although the above studies had shown that folic acid can reduce the incidence of NTDs, the Food and Drug Administration (FDA) had not approved this intervention, nor had the CDC issued recommendations for the use of folic acid as a means of prevention. Their positions stemmed from the concern that the use of folic acid might mask the detection of pernicious anemia. Additionally, it was not clear whether the scientific evidence was strong enough to make a public health recommendation. Citing the pernicious anemia risk, the National Institutes of Health (NIH) believed that additional research was needed. We believed that doing nothing represented the greatest risk.

Meanwhile, Cameron County residents accused us of diverting attention from the real issue, namely, poor environmental conditions. They felt we should conduct more water, soil, and air testing to determine the exact cause of defects. They feared that if the focus shifted from causation to prevention, the greater issue of health and environmental concerns would once again be ignored, and citizens would be left helpless and defenseless against environmental risks such as unregulated industrial activities, pesticide use, and lack of sanitation facilities.

While we had no intention of ending the search for the cause of NTDs in South Texas, we agreed that ignoring the information accumulating about folic acid would be tantamount to malpractice. Promoting folic acid would allow us to be proactive in reducing the risk of birth defects and to offer some hope to young families. Thus, the TDH took the lead in promoting the use of folic acid, ahead of the CDC and the FDA. We prayed that we were right and launched an aggressive educational campaign. At the same time, we worked through a long FDA approval process with the CDC, NIH, and FDA in order to issue a health claim acknowledging folic acid as an effective tool against anencephaly, spina bifida, and other NTDs. Our suggestions were eventually embraced, and in September 1992, the CDC published recommendations on folic acid consumption for American women of childbearing age. Later, a summit was held in the Lower Rio Grande Valley, where an international group of experts examined findings from Hungary, England, and Canada corroborating the use of folic acid.

Starting a campaign to publicize folic acid meant making many decisions with little guidance. For folic acid to be successful in preventing NTDs, a woman needs to have adequate levels of it in her system prior to pregnancy and during the first 28 days after conception. But most women do not know they are pregnant at this stage. Our challenge was to convince women to use folic acid before they conceived. Our message also had to explain to women how they could get the recommended dosage. There are three ways to ingest folic acid: through foods that naturally contain high levels of folic acid, through foods fortified with folic acid, and with a multivitamin supplement. We decided the easiest way to ensure adequate daily consumption of folic acid was to recommend taking a multivitamin. Additionally, the multivitamin would also provide other nutrients women needed during pregnancy. The National Scientific Advisory Committee supported our decision to promote multivitamins, recognizing that asking women to rely on careful dietary planning for the proper daily dosage of folic acid would be difficult and even impractical over time. This is why Texas was the first state to advocate fortifying staple foods with folic acid.

The health promotion staff of the TDH developed an educational program for health care professionals and public audiences on NTDs and on taking folic acid to prevent them. Local providers were asked for input. The program included a toll-free information line for materials, referrals, and additional information; a scripted slide show for health care providers and their staff; and printed guidelines for women of childbearing age. In March 1993, the TDH awarded a grant to an advertising agency to develop a media campaign and poster in English and Spanish. The resulting advertisements were aired statewide. Narrated by women with babies, the advertisements encourage all women of childbearing age to take multivitamins with folic acid. The campaign slogan was, "Before you start making a baby, start taking multivitamins with folic acid." As far as we know, this was the first time in the United States that advertising had been used to promote taking folic acid in multivitamin form as a weapon against NTDs. Another unique aspect of the campaign was that it was funded with contributions from pharmaceutical companies.

The combined efforts of the companies and the health department show how business and government can work together to effectively address health concerns.

In addition to informing providers and the public about the benefits of folic acid, the TDH offered free multivitamin and folic acid supplements to low-income women of childbearing age in Cameron and Hidalgo Counties. The vitamins were donated by pharmaceutical companies. Since the program's inception in October 1992, the TDH has overseen the distribution of over 145,000 bottles of multivitamins to an estimated 45,000 women of childbearing age.

SYSTEMS CHANGES

Because of our commitment to the people of Cameron County and the collaborative effort among state and federal agencies and private companies, we have improved conditions along the border. Most notably, the TDH successfully advocated for two critical pieces of legislation affecting the border. One established a state registry for birth defects with yearly appropriations of $3 million; the other created the Office of Border Environmental and Consumer Health.

The NTD crisis in Cameron County highlighted the need for a formal statewide monitoring system for all birth defects. A birth defects registry facilitates the identification of birth defect clusters through accurate and ongoing incidence evaluation, trend analysis, cluster identification, and etiologic investigation. Data can be shared and compared with other states, possibly leading to strategies for the prevention of birth defects.

The attitude encountered during the 73rd session of the Texas legislature was one of fiscal conservatism. Legislators were not very receptive to new programs or those requiring additional general revenue. Advocacy and community groups such as the March of Dimes and Children's Defense Fund worked with us to reach the legislature with our message. Our strategy was to make heart-wrenching truths known:

- Annually more than 12,000 Texas children are born with birth defects, accounting for 25 percent of infant deaths.
- Birth defects caused by alcohol, cocaine, seizure medication, and folic acid deficiency are preventable.
- Many of the infants who survive face a lifetime of chronic disability and illness and cost their families and the state millions of dollars.
- If birth defects were prevented in only eight children, the birth defects registry would pay for itself.

After the law was enacted, pilot programs for the birth defects registry were initiated in the Rio Grande Valley and the Houston area. During the 74th Legislative Session, lawmakers approved $1 million in additional money, enabling the TDH to expand the registry so that it covered 75 percent of Texas cities the following year. The National Scientific Advisory Committee was reconfigured to become the advisory committee for the new registry.

The legislation creating the Office of Border Environmental and Consumer Health has allowed us to maintain a strong presence in the valley. This office works with health services and providers to address health concerns. The office oversees border field staff who are experts in environmental engineering, toxicology, epidemiology, sanitation, and food safety.

There have been other significant successes since we initiated our activities. The CDC has issued recommendations urging women of childbearing age to increase their intake of folic acid. The fruits of a long and intensive education campaign to promote the fortification of corn meal and flour were realized on February 29, 1996, when the FDA formally recommended using folic acid as a supplement in corn meal, bread, and flour.

Texas and Mexico health officials have developed a method to better understand NTDs on both sides of the border, including an agreement on a standard assessment methodology for both the United States and Mexico. In October 1992, Texas was one of two states awarded a CDC-funded, five-year cooperative agreement of more than $300,000 per year for expanded NTD surveillance, educational activities, intervention with folic acid, and evaluation of risk factors in the 14 counties along the Texas-Mexico border. To date, the project has enabled approximately 50 women who previously suffered the pain of giving birth to a child with an NTD to give birth to a healthy infant after taking folic acid. The case-control study that is underway as part of this agreement will give us our best chance yet to unravel the mystery of NTDs.

Although these accomplishments represent major breakthroughs for the agency and scientific community, I am proudest of the fact that the NTD crisis forced national attention on the long-neglected health and environmental issues of the Texas-Mexico border. As a result, significant resources are being directed to this underserved community to enhance the health status of its residents. For example, because of water sampling efforts that began during our initial investigation, several waterways in the Lower Rio Grande Valley have been closed to fishing for health reasons. While an environmental cause for NTDs has not been found, our efforts have brought further attention to the hazards of pesticides and polychlorobiphenyls (PCBs) in and around the colonies.

REFLECTIONS

Out of this crisis came opportunity. This was a period of personal turmoil and growth, and listening became my predominant activity. Direct communication with those concerned and its consequence—relaying a broader health message—became our best offense. Second guessing by local officials and national experts kept us challenged and on task. A multifaceted and integrated scientific approach to explaining the high incidence of NTDs and an aggressive policy to prevent them did away with some of the local community's confusion and mistrust. Because we invited assistance outside of government—both state and federal—we were able to validate and sell our strategy. A solid game plan with achievable goals gave us all an opportunity to celebrate. Curiosity and science ultimately guided our decisions, but we never forgot that axiom of the ages: All politics are local.

PART III

Local Health Agencies in Transition

CHAPTER 6

Toward a Population Focus: The Transition of a Local Health Department

Thomas L. Milne

Like many local health departments in the United States, the S.W. Washington Health District invested many of its resources in health services for individuals in the 1980s and early 1990s. In recent years, most of the health district's activities have targeted individuals rather than populations. As executive director of the organization, I had concerns about our focus on personal health services. I believed, for example, that we were losing opportunities to leverage our limited resources to provide broader prevention services. On the other hand, I shared staff concerns about the limited availability and accessibility of clinical services for the low income clients we were serving with our programs. Passage of the Washington State Health Services Act of 1993, however, made it clear to me that the public health services had to change to complement rather than augment the privately based, capitated, managed health care system of the future.

The S.W. Washington Health District serves three counties in the southwest corner of Washington State. Clark County is urban, with a rapidly growing population of 305,000. Skamania and Klickitat counties are small and rural, with populations of 9,500 and 18,500, respectively. Currently the health district has a budget of $10 million, employs about 190 staff members, and is governed by a board of health that consists of 13 elected city and county officials.

THE TASK AT HAND

It was apparent early in Washington State's 1993 legislative session that health reform would become a reality. A two-year study conducted by the prestigious Health Care Commission resulted in legislation that was comprehensive in approach and boasted broad bipartisan and bicameral support. Under the act, competing managed care systems, paid through capitation, would provide a health package with specified benefits to all residents within seven years. Strengthening the public health infrastructure was a core element of the legislation, with revenue allocation to be determined in 1994 after the Public Health Improvement Plan (PHIP) was completed, as called for by legislation. The intended purpose of PHIP was to identify core capacities (for which the state and local health departments would be held accountable), current capacities, and the resources needed to achieve full capacity statewide.

It was clear that PHIP and legislated changes in the health care system would have a huge impact on local public health departments. How would we transform the role and structure of the health district when we were faced with so many unknowns? My goal was to reconfigure the services offered in the district. The new structure would complement the new health care system, maximize our contribution to the communities we serve, and in the future meet the PHIP capacity standards that were being developed. I also wanted to make sure that our health department would continue to play a critical role in the context of the changing delivery system. To achieve this goal, I concluded that it was essential to involve four key groups: the board of health, staff members, the union, and leaders among the provider community.

The Board of Health

If the restructuring was to be successful, it was critical that board members understood the need for change and supported the reform. My board of health directs policy for Clark, Skamania, and Klickitat counties. Each of the 13 board members is an elected official who represents the interests of one of the counties or towns and cities in the district. Although each member tries to keep the big picture in mind when deliberating on board of health matters, member allegiances and priorities rest with the city, town, or county each represents. As executive director I didn't expect opposition to needed changes. Nonetheless, it was clear that my biggest challenge would be making sure that the board considered differences in provider systems and resident needs in each of the three counties.

Staff Members

New directions would not be taken without the board's approval; however, changes could not be adequately planned or implemented without the involvement and support of staff. I was confident that my management team would understand the need for change and would participate fully in defining the new directions health departments would take. In 1993 my management team comprised a physician health officer and four division directors. We met weekly, working closely to develop policy, to plan budgets, and to oversee operations. The level of trust and mutual respect is very high among team members.

Management leadership is joined by supervisors and operations coordinators in monthly meetings to discuss trends and operational issues. I expected the group to understand the changing environment of contemporary health care, to participate in making decisions, and to help inform staff about the reforms we decided to implement. General staff comprise the largest segment of health district personnel. I expected resistance to the significant changes we wanted to make if staff did not receive frequent and accurate information about the changes.

Union Members

The union was the third key group to consider. All nonexempt staff belong to a single labor union. A business manager, who is an employee of the union, represents the union, and I expected him to resist changes that might jeopardize the continued employment of union members or that might challenge worker rights.

Over the years, we have developed an excellent working relationship with the union. We use collaborative or "win-win" approaches in our collective bargaining, and we have formed two labor-and-management committees to deal with contract and noncontract issues before serious problems arise. The success of our relationship is demonstrated in part by ongoing, amicable relations: We have experienced only one staff grievance in the past five years. Accordingly, I believed that the union representative would support the organizational changes if he understood the rationale behind them and if he was assured that the changes took into account the individual needs of staff members.

Health Care Leaders

The fourth key group comprised leaders from the medical community. The principal players in this group were the administrator of the S.W. Washington Medical Center in Clark County and the director of Community Affairs for Kaiser Permanente, Northwest Region. The chief executive officer (CEO) of the medical center was chair of the state hospital association and had served as a member of the Health Care Commission. He clearly understood the importance of maintaining a healthy community in the context of capitated managed care. I expected him to support changes that would help his organization contain costs by promoting health care on a population level, and I hoped that he would provide assistance to the health district to support reform. Similarly, the Kaiser Permanente community affairs director understood that her organization needed to invest in population-level prevention to improve health status and contain costs. I expected her to support changes in the health district that would contribute to Kaiser Permanente's interests: the improvement of the health of enrollees. It was difficult to identify leadership among the physician groups. I expected that some would be concerned with the economic impact of assuming responsibility for low income patients who would no longer be served by the health district as change progressed.

Change was inevitable. The Health Services Act had passed, and I was beginning to sense that change was occurring in the local health care system. Moreover, PHIP was about to be implemented. As we began planning our organization's restructuring, I viewed the major health care providers in the community as potential sources of support. I felt that the biggest challenge would be to find the best fit between the needs of the health district and those services provided by new health care systems. I was also interested in bringing staff, the union, and members of the board together to facilitate reform.

STRATEGIES AND TACTICS

In early 1993 I met with my management team to discuss ideas about the changing environment of local health care and to begin a planning process. Members of the team expressed strong concerns about the impact of anticipated changes in the delivery of health care, both in terms of quality and access to care. My colleagues agreed with my initial assessment that significant changes in our role were inevitable. Together we developed strategies to address the challenges we were facing. Although the issues considered in each of the three counties were similar, change would affect Clark County first. For the sake of brevity, I will describe our plans and their results in Clark County only.

Strategy 1: Define What the Local Health Care Delivery System Will Look Like

To define the role that we would play, we first needed to understand what changes the local provider system would make in response to the Health Services Act. In early 1993, there was a serious shortage of physicians in Clark County, which is mostly urban. Only one hospital/medical center was located there. Local physicians participated in a variety of Oregon-based health plans. Managed care arrangements served about 40 percent of county residents, mostly through Kaiser Permanente. It was expected that several of Portland's hospital-based managed care systems were preparing to provide services in Clark County. Although our relationships with the local providers were good, we were not well informed of their plans to address provider shortages, issues in managed care, or external competition.

We decided to participate more closely with the medical center and with Kaiser Permanente. We wanted to learn how those organizations saw their evolving roles, and we also wanted to take part in their development to the extent that public health concerns were involved. Toward this end, we held regular meetings with the executive officer of the medical center, with members of the provider systems, and with physician groups. We engaged in discussions of issues such as system capacity, provider recruitment, reorganization efforts, interests in population-level prevention, and community assessment. We also recognized that a communitywide assessment and the strategic planning process for a healthier Clark County were important elements in this strategy.

Other tactics presented themselves. For example, I was asked to become a member of the medical center's board of trustees in early 1994. In response, I expressed my concern that I would be expected to participate in advocating for policies that were in the interest of the center and not in the interest of the community as a whole. The board chairman replied, "That's what we want from you, Tom—advocacy for the health of the entire community." Given such a response, I decided to join the board, and consequently I have had an opportunity to participate in discussions and help shape policy about the changing function of the medical center.

Strategy 2: Define the Future Role, Function, and Organization of the Health District

The future of the health district depends not only on the private sector but also on our changing revenue streams, the then-to-be-developed provisions of PHIP, and the preferences of our local board of health. Taking these factors into consideration, the management team decided on a variety of tactics. These included involving staff in the development of a shared vision, aggressive forecasting of future revenue streams, incorporating PHIP principles and guidelines as they evolved, making frequent presentations to the board of health, arranging an all-day retreat to help the board make decisions, and maintaining communications with staff to keep them current with the thinking and planning as it occurred.

Strategy 3: Defer Significant Revenue Loss

As we began our planning in 1993, the state Medicaid agency decided to effect a transition from fee-for-service payments to managed care. The agency agreed to allow local health departments to continue billing for some services for up to two years after the start-up of the managed care program. We were told that managed Medicaid services would begin in Clark County in January 1994.

Our 1993 operating revenues included $766,000 in clinical revenues from Medicaid; however, it was difficult to project what to expect in 1994 and beyond. Variables included the pace of enrollment; the percentage of former clients who were still eligible to receive our services, but who would now choose to use services from the managed care system in which they enrolled; and the speed with which that shift took place.

To ensure a smooth transition, we planned methods to defer significant revenue loss. Our tactics included forecasting revenue, identifying vulnerable services and staff, and developing short, intermediate, and long-term plans describing health district services and staffing.

Strategy 4: Ensure that Staff Members, the Union, and the Board of Health Participate in the Changes

I have identified this strategy as separate even though the other three stratagems actively incorporated the participation of these groups. I believe that it is of the greatest importance to keep staff fully informed of and, when possible, involved in the change process. Even when change is planned and those affected understand it, the experience can be frightening. When significant reform in an organization occurs and includes changes in job assignment, the changes can be paralyzing, especially when planned "in the dark." Moreover, it was clear that the excellent working relationship between union and management would be quickly jeopardized if the rationale behind the change was not carefully communicated. Finally, even the most reasoned and carefully planned transition, brought about by the best of staff, would go nowhere if the governing board didn't agree to the reforms. It was critical that the board of health be prepared, with a well-thought-out policy framework provided by management.

We employed several tactics to keep staff apprised of our thinking. To promote communication, we published an internal, staff-generated newsletter incorporating a monthly column that I wrote, as well as staff meetings, yearly all-staff retreats, brown bag meetings, and informal discussions at divisional and team levels. I met regularly with the union business manager, and we incorporated concerns that we couldn't previously resolve into our 1994 collective bargaining process. I provided monthly updates to the full board on the progress of our planning. In the summer of 1994, we also scheduled a full-day retreat for the board. At this retreat, we asked the board to respond formally to policy changes we developed to guide our transition.

Strategy 5: Implement Organizational Change To Position the Health District for the Future

We planned to use the results of the other four strategies to define needed organizational changes and the timing of their implementation. We agreed on meeting the principal PHIP capacity standards when they went into effect in July 1995. Our tactics included the following:

- developing organizational principles consistent with our vision and changing environment;
- identifying internal opportunities for shifts in resources to population-focused services;
- analyzing private sector service availability and capacity for personal health services provided by the health district; and
- exploring options to replace clinical with population-focused services, a change reflecting the core public health capacities defined by PHIP.

WHAT HAPPENED

We pursued the first four strategies concurrently, and organizational changes were made when the timing was right. Tactics were often modified as we made progress with a particular strategy. I assigned lead responsibility for several of the core tactics to members of our management team, and we monitored progress together on a monthly and sometimes weekly basis in team meetings.

Local Health Delivery System

Our efforts at characterizing the evolving local provider system have been very successful, owing in large part to our greater inclusion of the medical center's board of trustees and in our establishing provider planning sessions. The community assessment and strategic planning process we began in 1993 opened several doors, giving us a clearer picture of both the health needs in the county and the provider system's changing capacity and structure. Through my participation as a medical center trustee, I have had opportunities to contribute to planning and policy development from a public health perspective. Due in part to my advocacy, the medical center and Kaiser Permanente each contributed $50,000, both in 1995 and again in 1996, to support implementation of the community project, Community Choices 2010. This project, which was the product of the community assessment and strategic planning project we initiated, is mobilizing residents to create a healthier Clark County.

As somewhat of a surprise, the state legislature eliminated several key provisions of the Health Services Act in 1995. Undaunted, the medical center CEO continued to move this organization and the physician community in the direction of a physician-hospital-community organization (PHCO). Increasing competition was the motivating force behind his efforts. More than 60 percent of county residents now receive their medical care through managed care organizations, and the numbers are growing rapidly. As it develops, the PHCO will invest in improving the county's health status and will help to assure access to health care for all county residents. The medical center CEO believes that the greatest potential for true health care reform is not at the federal or state level but at the local level.

The medical center initiated a family practice residency program in 1995. The program is intended not only to provide excellent training for primary care physicians but also to increase the number of such physicians choosing Clark County to practice. Aggressive recruiting by the medical center and Kaiser Permanente have also contributed to a reduction in the physician shortage.

Our tactics to increase linkages with the provider community have also led to closer working relationships with physicians and their offices in a variety of practice areas, including immunization, human immunodeficiency virus (HIV) treatment and prevention activities, and the control of communicable diseases. We also offer family practice residents the chance to work in a public health rotation. We are receiving encouragement from Kaiser Permanente regarding access to Health Plan Employer Data and Information Set (HEDIS) and other outcome data. Seeking ways to further the district's capacity to provide prevention activities at a population level, Kaiser Permanente has requested our input in the design of a new facility in Clark County.

In short, our work on developing a clearer picture of changes occurring in the health care delivery system was successful and resulted in significantly improved linkages between various elements of the system.

Bringing the Board Along

As board members watched changes in the health system develop, they began to understand fully the urgency behind the messages I had been giving. At our retreat in 1994, board members considered policy options developed by the management team regarding core services, financing, and governance. Concerns expressed at a board meeting two years earlier about the need to "protect the safety net" were replaced with directions to leverage the health district's resources to improve health status. We got the "go ahead" to proceed with the transition.

Bringing Staff Along: Shared Vision

In 1992–1993, I participated in the first Public Health Leadership Institute. I chose for my "learning project" the development of a shared vision in the health district. Building on ideas originating in a staff retreat a couple of years earlier, in late 1993 I led our management group in drafting a vision statement reflecting recent changes in our environment. We used the draft to help guide planning during 1994.

I met with small groups of staff between February and May 1995, spending about 45 minutes with each group. I began the sessions by discussing changes in the organization of local health services and in funding services. We also discussed the implications of PHIP, which had been adopted by the 1995 state legislature. I explained that shared vision statements describe an organization's desired future by incorporating the views of all members of the organization. I added that these statements serve as one of the principal foundations of an organization, along with mission and values statements. We concluded the sessions with a 15-minute writing assignment, during which staff considered their operational environment, the draft vision statement written in 1993, and what they believed the health district should look like in the future. Responses were varied: Some edited the draft statement, some wrote only a few words, and some wrote for 20 minutes. But all contributed.

Next I appointed a small committee of line staff and managers, asking them to organize all the staff members' written contributions and extract the essence of their statements in order to fashion a succinct vision statement. The committee produced an excellent shared vision statement and presented it during a staff retreat in October 1995, where it was received to a standing ovation. To communicate our ideas to the public, we hung two posters throughout our seven facilities. One included staff contributions by category, while the other offered our health district's shared vision statement.

Deferring Revenue Loss and Bringing the Union Along: A Convergence

Perhaps the most challenging of our problems was determining when the changes in revenue would occur and how much our revenue would drop. The forecasts for Medicaid revenues we made in 1994 quickly proved to be far too optimistic. The implementation of a new, managed Medicaid reimbursement structure was brought about more efficiently than we had projected, and our former clients began seeking services from their new primary care physicians more quickly than we had expected. As we entered labor negotiations in March 1994, projections indicated that we were headed for a revenue shortfall in excess of $400,000 for the year, with continued losses in the first six months of 1995. We were expecting a significant influx of new funds from PHIP in July 1995, so we considered the problem temporary.

Working collaboratively with the union, we developed a strategy to avoid or minimize layoffs. Collectively, we decided on the following actions, which would be used serially, as needed: (1) We would search for new revenue sources, (2) we would offer voluntary furloughs, and (3) we would reduce hours for *all* union and management staff, including myself. If these charges didn't solve the fiscal problem, we agreed that layoffs would then occur.

Initially, I hoped that financial assistance would come from the medical center and Kaiser Permanente. Leaders of both organizations were concerned that the health district's transition in providing broader prevention services would be interrupted. The medical center CEO offered financial assistance, and we were examining options when my clinic services director discovered that one of our existing revenue streams, Federal Medicaid Administrative Match (FMAM), had the potential to provide additional income. The revenues we generated from FMAM more than covered our actual shortfall. Although the assistance ultimately wasn't needed, the offer from the CEO underlined both the importance of the changing focus of the health district to the medical center and our improving relationship.

Both the union and staff were very pleased with management's pledge to share in reduction of hours and recognized how successful management's efforts were in eliminating the shortfall. We are still facing serious fiscal concerns today, however. PHIP revenues are significantly less than what had been projected, and we expect FMAM funds to be sharply reduced or eliminated through the welfare reform actions of Congress. I explained to the board the importance of deferring additional revenue losses as long as possible to assure completion of our organization's transition, which will be completed in 1998. In response to our concerns, the board approved the establishment of a transition fund, based on the increase in FMAM income. The monies will be spent down as revenue reductions occur. This decision was made even as the Clark County commissioners, all three of whom are board of health members, were making reductions in other internal programs to balance their budget.

Changes in the Organization

By the end of 1994, we had developed organizational models for July 1995 (the date of PHIP's implementation), for 1997, and for 2000. By the end of 1995, we had nearly completed the transition planning process and had made a number of significant organizational changes. Relatively early, we incorporated our maternity services program into a new nurse-midwife–based maternity program at the medical center. Additionally, we moved our diabetes education and cardiovascular risk programs to medical center sponsorship.

Recognizing that the provider community offers a broader base of services, we have eliminated our well and sick baby clinics, school dental services, a mobile school clinic, and travel clinics. Client access to most of these services has been assured, either through service contracts, funded in part with health district funds, or through provider agreements to assume responsibility. At present, we are working with stakeholders and other providers in the community to determine continuing access to women's reproductive health, refugee and immigration health, general clinic, and clinical laboratory services.

We have reduced staff-provided immunizations by over 60 percent by distributing vaccines to provider offices rather than directly offering immunizations. Through the vaccine distribution program, staff is given entry into private clinics and practices. There they provide training to office staff, set up quality assurance programs, and help develop procedures for following up patients. In addition, staff have developed partnerships with local physicians, businesses, and others to implement highly visible programs providing immunizations to the community. Even though the health district has reduced the number of vaccines directly administered, the quality and attainment of immunization levels in Clark County have *risen* overall as a direct result of our population focus.

Program eliminations and reductions do not comprise all of the changes in the health district. Additionally, we have created a deputy director position, set up an urgent needs response team, combined clinical and community health divisions, started a Center for Assessment, Planning and Evaluation (CAPE), and made major improvements in the health district's local area network (LAN)-based information system. Throughout these changes, we have maintained our commitment to honor our most important resource: our staff. With the exception of the deputy director, existing staff have filled all of the new positions. Two nurse practitioners wishing to remain clinicians were assisted in finding positions in private practices; only one nurse practitioner was laid off.

As we effect our transition to more broadly based population services, our credibility is dependent on our ability to deliver high-quality services. To accommodate the many significant changes occurring in staff responsibilities, I asked the board to approve a significant increase in funding for staff training. During 1995, over half of our staff received training in the core functions of public health. Another 30 staff members completed a course on the basics of community assessment, which included material on biostatistics and epidemiology. Our CAPE staff received intensive training in biostatistics, computer modeling, and related areas. We plan to implement a staff development program in 1997.

The new deputy director is responsible for formalizing the policy development process and for providing information to the public. Together, we are working with the medical center and a local university to establish a center for health policy. The deputy director has designed a framework for policy development and works closely with the director of CAPE to assure that policy development activities in the health district are linked to assessment outcomes. After the health district created CAPE in January 1995 to institutionalize community assessment, the director and four CAPE staff members completed a community assessment in Skamania and Klickitat counties later in the same year. Both these assessments were tied to strategic planning efforts. In 1996 CAPE updated the Clark County assessment that was completed in 1993 and completed an environmental health assessment. The team has also created evaluation methodologies for reviewing internal programs.

Our urgent needs team includes public health nursing, environmental health, and health education staff along with clerical support. The team, directed by the deputy director, was created to address developing public health issues, using innovative approaches to provide population level health services. Convening the team was also our first effort at setting up a self-managing work group, a concept we wish to explore for future organizing of services.

All changes in the organization are consistent with our shared vision and have enabled us to fulfill the capacity standards of PHIP. By July 1995, we had met our goal of becoming a turnkey organization; fully operational units now provided community assessment, mobilization, and population-focused prevention activities. Our improved linkages with providers increased our capacity to assure access to services.

Bringing Staff and the Union Along

Keeping staff and the union aware of changes throughout the process required vigilance. Their informed contribution was and continues to be a critically important element of our transition. Our joint labor-management committee meets monthly and discusses rumors, communication issues, staff morale, and workplace problems. It is true that rumors develop in our organization, as happens everywhere, but most don't survive long, owing to work of the committee. When changes encroach on provisions of the labor contract, the labor-management committee deals with contractual issues to head off conflict. The work of both committees is shared openly with all staff. Finally, I meet with the staff association monthly and regularly attend division or program meetings to provide updates on changes in the organization.

CONCLUSION

At this point, I am very pleased with our work and would change little. Although there have been no road maps and little external assistance to help us find the way, we have effectively changed our organization. My leadership role throughout the transition has been to assure that both our planning and our information were sound, that community leaders and our board understood both the rationale behind the transition and its general direction, and that we kept to our task. I have also tried to help our management team and other participants within our organization build on the inventions and discoveries we have made together along the way. Much of the insight and innovation, and most of the work of the transition, was done by my managers, a wonderfully skilled and highly empowered group of public health professionals.

We have completed the requisite shift in our thinking about the health district's role in the communities we serve, and we have seen that shift in outlook occur from the management team through most staff. Our new values hold that the health district's highest contributions to the community will be achieved through the provision of population-level services, including community assessment, policy development through community mobilization, population-focused health promotion and prevention, and the assurance of access and quality in community-based services. Those values further hold that personal clinical services are best provided in a system managed by the private sector. The changing provider system will remove disincentives for providers to care for the poor while providing alternative entry points to overcome barriers to access. Our role revision best complements the health care provider system currently evolving in Clark County. We are fortunate to have a provider community that agrees.

In a recent demonstration that locally assured universal access is more than a dream, the medical center and Kaiser Permanente requested that I both facilitate and participate in a series of meetings intended to identify means of providing care for the indigent. At the first meeting, we broadened our goals to find a way of providing care for all Clark County residents, as well as improving the health status of county residents.

I believe that most of the changes we have made at the health district are irreversible. Much of our core capacity to provide clinical services has been lost, and so we are dependent upon the private provider system for their provision. But most of the capacity loss would have occurred even if we had made no changes, because Medicaid, the principal revenue source for our clinical services, moved to finance services through managed care systems. My moment of significant alarm occurred when the health reform act was eviscerated by the state legislature in 1995. Local providers have continued to offer care, however, and local commitment to universal access is as strong as ever.

I have not addressed in this chapter the changes planned for environmental health services, but we anticipate several. CAPE included environmental issues in the Skamania and Klickitat assessments. Its environmental health assessment in Clark County added a set of community strategies to the Community Choices 2010 strategic plan.

In conclusion, we are positioning our organization to respond to the future and believe that we will be much more effective in improving the health of the community once we leverage our assets and form partnerships with community organizations.

CHAPTER 7

Public Health Leadership in DeKalb County

Paul J. Wiesner

In 1989, when I was interviewed for my current position, the questions asked by members of the DeKalb County Board of Health suggested that they wanted a combination of things: a manager, a person with good technical skills, and someone who would get along well with others.

Nowhere in the interview process did we discuss my passion for social justice, my commitment to making some sense out of the jumble of categorical public health efforts, or my deeply felt enthusiasm for public health's broad mission, as articulated by the report that the Institute of Medicine (IOM) had recently issued on the future of public health. It was clear that the board was not obtuse and that I was not deceptive. Pursuing a transforming vision just didn't seem of major importance.

To me, the IOM report meant the following: Public health is not what the health department does, but what we all do individually and collectively to create the conditions in which people can be healthy. At each new employee orientation I emphasized the "three Cs": caring, competence, and connections. Our employees heard about the three Cs regularly, because I made a practice of visiting every new employee at the monthly get-togethers. I envisioned a continuous connection between our agency and the people we served, group participation in decisions that helped us to be healthy, and a sense of caring for one another. The professional public health practitioner brought technical expertise and information to the table, and the community brought wisdom, insight, and energy. Working together with mutual respect, we could make our county healthier.

But when I arrived at the DeKalb County Board of Health, its mission was quite different. The staff and programs of the Board of Health had an excellent reputation for providing high quality personal preventive services in a clinical setting. But what we now call "core" population-based services, that is, essential public health activities, were not central either to the cultural lore or to the practice of decision making at the DeKalb County Board of Health. The data, when organized, were used to direct clinical services. The focus was on professional, medically related activities rather than on the community and its lay leaders. Care was greatly influenced by the mental health section of the agency, whose specific statutory mandate was to serve the neediest people suffering from mental illness, mental retardation, and substance addictions. As a result of these influences, our staff emphasized services to those most in need. Promotion of wellness and health, policy development, surveillance, epidemiology, and broad community collaboration were all secondary to the provision of individual personal services to the "needy."

The story of transforming public health in DeKalb County is not about responding to an external threat or about meeting a specific crisis. Rather, it is about a group of people, some of them agency veterans and some of them new like myself, working to take on a subtle challenge. In our particular circumstances, a successful changeover in the public health services could best be built on the Board of Health's existing strengths. I suppose that is always the case, but it seemed extremely important to acknowledge the excellence of services when we were dealing with an agency that already had a very good reputation. Our problem—maybe it would be better described as our opportunity—was to effect a shift in the thinking and the behavior of an agency that saw itself as very effective, and to do so even though there was not a perceived threat from the outside.

We sought to move the emphasis from supplying personal services to individuals, particularly those deemed "most-in-need," to the broader mission of providing essential services to the whole community. I believed then, and still believe six years later, that if our agency had continued with the paradigm that had worked so well for it in the past, it would have died a slow death, and the real potential of public health to provide a broad spectrum of care would never have been realized in my county. Great opportunities for improved health status would have been lost. I intuitively concluded that we needed to do the opposite of the old adage, "If it ain't broke, don't fix it." We *had* to break accepted practices in order to fix them, to transform them for the future. Acting as the leader rather than as the manager of the agency, I was forced to ask how I might begin to transform what we were then into that which we needed to become.

It was often impossible for me to know whose ideas were whose as our efforts unfolded. In my own mind, it is very clear that none of our progress would have occurred without a team approach involving a very talented and dedicated staff, the support of the board, and a very strong tradition in our county of working together in many spheres. Everything that was accomplished was done by many people working in concert. Every strategy developed, every tactic executed, and certainly every success (and failure) resulted because a group of people worked together in this transformation. In fact, even those resisting change contributed because they wanted to preserve what was good in the organization.

Because we had a number of key senior people who were cautious, effective managers of our fiscal and programmatic efforts, I had the luxury of pursuing a vision of change. In addition, the concept I started out with was general and incompletely formulated. That vision certainly changed over time, particularly under the influence of people like Dr. Lawrence Sanders, who eventually became deputy director of the agency. Drs. Joyce Essien and Jane Nelson, from Emory University's Rollins School of Public Health, also provided a valuable perspective and impetus for refining the ideas and developing improved strategies for implementing our organizational changes.

Our attempts to transform the DeKalb County Board of Health and its relationship to the people we serve and to others who have an interest in what we do in the county met with criticism, concerns, substantial confusion, and, occasionally, intense conflict. For some, the idea of change meant that I had made a definitive negative judgment about the status quo. For these people, change was indicated only when something major was wrong. They knew that they maintained the status quo, and they feared that any change represented a negative assessment of them, of their worth, and of their performance.

The vision required to accomplish this transformation was seen by others, at times, to conflict with the agency's need to maintain solid fiscal and programmatic management. We had our share of practical problems that could have easily occupied much of my time and energy. Because my management style is open, people had more information. For that reason, however, old issues that had been smoldering rose more readily to the surface. As a result, the daily chores of management increased in number and complexity. The temptation to focus my energies on resolving internal problems was great. Pursuing a vision often seemed frivolous and maybe even foolhardy in light of the daily practical challenges.

There was also the institutional inertia that occurs naturally in an organization, a relatively large one of 1,000 employees. About 60 percent of our resources were devoted to the Division of Mental Health, Mental Retardation and Substance Abuse, which had a very strong traditional mandate to serve those individuals who were most in need in the community. I realized that it would be very difficult to realize our vision of serving the whole community when so many of our resources were devoted to a very small population segment. The initial challenges—fear of change, conflict between pursuing the vision and dealing with daily problems, and inertia—were daunting.

As we started to make changes, and as they were recognized as serious and real in nature, additional conflicts arose. Our team pursued reform in a very public way, incorporating marketing and public relations skills, and there was a concern that our efforts were merely "politics" and grandstanding. It was even suggested that my leadership was partly an ego trip. As a result, some questioned the substance of our effort. Additionally, staff in some of our fellow county agencies and departments demonstrated jealousy.

INITIAL STEPS

To obtain an assessment of the agency's strengths and areas for improvement, I visited more than 100 DeKalb county residents who were outside the agency. I asked them what they thought of the local Board of Health and what we could do to improve our performance. I purposefully kept the discussion general, and so each question was open-ended. During these hour-long discussions, I learned a lot about our county and our agency. I learned that while our reputation was good, our visibility was low. As a result of my talks and my own impressions, I came to believe that we had some critical requirements. We needed a vision and a larger constituency, we needed to shift our focus from "the most in need" to "the most to benefit," and we needed to broaden our base of resources and support.

Since I wanted the provisions of public health services in DeKalb County to be a true community venture, instead of focusing on the agency, I decided to focus on the community. My management team and I decided to try to go beyond the agency itself, to get out into the community and make our purpose known. We hoped to involve our agency with the community in such a way that the community would become the teacher and the agency the student. So, having decided on our game plan, we began our strategy of reaching the community. First, I accepted every chance I could to speak to community groups, often in forums or before breakfast clubs. At these meetings I repeated the three linchpins of my 10-year goal at the DeKalb County Board of Health: to establish a democratic procedure in making decisions about health, to rediscover ways of maintaining prevention and primary care, and to come to grips with the limits of our collective resources. I shared data about the health status of our community and in this way informed people about what was truly occurring. We made decisions together with lay persons.

We changed our focus: Instead of targeting communities with severe needs, we identified geographic areas offering an opportunity for prevention services. With the shift in emphasis I was trying to correct an abiding problem in public health practice, namely, the myth that if we describe the problem very precisely by the usual epidemiological parameters, more than half the battle is won. Unfortunately, such an analysis stigmatizes the relatively small group described in these evaluations, and as a result the group is separated from the resources that form the basis for improvement in health status.

Further, the public health problem-oriented approach has a negative ring to it. Instead, seeking to emphasize the positive, we first published a report on the status of the county's health, with the subtitle "Opportunities for Prevention and Community Service." Even though the geographic areas we depicted as ready for prevention services included the "traditional high-risk," a phrase that, along with "targeting," we have banned from our discussions of health care, we were careful to draw the boundaries broadly so as to include community-based assets that could help our prevention efforts.

In fact, the focus on assets became another theme. I stated over and over again that we believed in asset-based empowerment rather than risk- or deficit-based betterment. For instance, we were as interested in finding out why most teenagers did not become pregnant as we were in finding out why others did. We were interested in learning what assets these teens and their peers had and how peer-mentor programs could help tap into that strength. For broader communities, we believed that they also had within themselves the means of improvement.

We maximized our use of print, radio, and television media to get the message out about community-oriented public health. We continually emphasized that the health status of our community was the responsibility of many sectors—businesses, religious institutions, community organizations, school systems, and public health agencies as well as individuals. We focused attention on successful ventures, always recognizing the success of others. We saw each encounter with a group or an individual as a recruitment opportunity for promoting public health. This attitude was basic but essential to our constituency development. We had to be persistent, positive, and patient. We had to truly believe that an informed and organized public would be able to contribute in a positive way to its own health status.

Not surprisingly, we found out that people like to participate. The achievements were heartening. Together, we passed the first countywide clean indoor air ordinance in the state of Georgia. People for Good Health, a group of approximately 200 volunteers, worked hard to educate DeKalb County residents. As a result, in the 1992 general election voters passed a $29.7 million bond referendum to improve the county's public health and mental health facilities. Another community group in DeKalb County, Our Status of Health (SOH), conducted a community-based survey and, using consensus-building techniques, established five leading prevention priorities: injuries, substance abuse (including tobacco), cancer, teenage pregnancy, and human immunodeficiency virus/acquired immunodeficiency syndrome (HIV/AIDS).

PUBLIC HEALTH AND ELECTED OFFICIALS

More detailed stories about our efforts will provide insight into our approach. First, our clean indoor air initiative highlights how influence between elected officials and the professional public health leader can be shared and put to good use. It was 1992, an election year, and County Commissioner Annie Collins had several good reasons to be concerned about the effects of tobacco smoke on health. Her ailing mother was suffering from a chronic condition that was aggravated by tobacco smoke. Collins was campaigning hard for the position of chief executive officer of the county, and one of her staunch supporters was a pharmaceutical sales manager who was a long-time leader in the local chapter of the American Cancer Society. His company sold nicotine patches to help people stop smoking, and he himself was significantly bothered by environmental tobacco smoke. Collins believed that our county would benefit from a strong ordinance requiring clean indoor air. She wanted this to be something more than a campaign stance. She needed a forum.

We worked with Collins's supporters and with antismoking advocates to launch an educational campaign on the benefits of keeping indoor air free of environmental tobacco smoke. At the conference that we helped organize to announce our campaign, I summarized the consequences of tobacco-related illness in DeKalb County and highlighted with graphic photographs the tobacco advertisements on billboards located close to schools in the area. Experts from the Centers for Disease Control and Prevention discussed the effects of environmental tobacco smoke on health and reported on the movement throughout the United States to establish effective local ordinances. Representatives from the medical society and the local chamber of commerce spoke in favor of an ordinance. As a result of our efforts, some 120 people saw Collins, a major contender for county chief executive officer, taking a strong stand for a healthy environment. All the other major contenders followed suit, with the result that the issue was placed on the county commission agenda.

This anecdote demonstrates how important timing is to successful change. Opportunities to make improvements in local health policies don't appear every day, and it is important to recognize them and capitalize on them when they occur. The public health sector must lend its scientific findings to enlightened elected officials' platforms.

Getting the issue on the agenda was only the first step. A second story illustrates another aspect of the public health leader's relationship with elected officials. In 1991, Manuel Maloof, the incumbent chief executive officer of the county who was finishing his last term, appointed a study committee to evaluate the impact of the proposed Clean Indoor Air Ordinance and to recommend revisions before the ordinance was given formal consideration by the County Commission. The draft ordinance had already received the endorsement of the Board of Health, the county medical society, and the local chapters of the voluntary health agencies. Maloof, a self-taught, second-generation, Lebanese restaurant and bar owner, was arguably the most powerful Democratic politician in the county. He did not favor the proposed ordinance, but he did appoint a balanced committee, chaired by the president of the chamber of commerce and with six other members: two businessmen representing small employers, a lawyer and former county commissioner with ties to the Tobacco Institute, an articulate community antismoking advocate, a state public health physician involved in cancer and tobacco control, and myself. There were four smokers and three nonsmokers on the panel.

At the packed work session before the vote on the committee's revised ordinance, Maloof asked me a series of questions. We went back and forth: "Dr. Wiesner, you are American aren't you?" I replied, "Yes, Mr. Chairman, I am an American." "Dr. Wiesner, you believe in freedom, don't you?" "You know I do, sir." "Don't you think that people are smart enough to vote with their feet and leave any place of business if the smoke is bothering them? Now, I think smoking is real bad for people, and on the advice of my doctor, I quit myself some time ago. But I don't believe in taking people's freedom away from them. It is one of the real treasures of being an American. Our freedom is sacred, don't you agree, Dr. Wiesner?" "I agree that our freedom is sacred. But in this country our citizens also have a right to petition their government to protect them from environmental toxins that cause cancer. Responsible people have put this ordinance up for your decision, and I certainly hope that this commission will vote 'Yes' on this one."

Three factors permitted me to engage Maloof in the manner I did. First, he was a fair man; I respected him and he knew that. Second, we had the scientific facts on our side. But third, and perhaps most important, we had built a constituency that respected our integrity and our commitment to making DeKalb County a healthier place.

PURSUING NEW GOALS

Nothing in my nearly seven years in local public health points more clearly to the importance of timing than our decision to pursue a bond referendum to build new health facilities. Since 1968, when the county government last built a new clinical health center, the population of our county has nearly doubled in size. By state law in Georgia, it is the responsibility of the county government to provide the facilities and equipment for the Board of Health's service programs. Because our facilities had not kept pace with the needs, our clinical services were offered in a series of embarrassingly old buildings and a few privately owned clinical centers, which were built to our specifications but required nearly one million dollars in rent each year. We see 20 percent of our population in our health centers, and some of our busiest clinics were the oldest and most rundown.

Some attention had been given to the sorry state of our physical facilities, but there was little action. In the late 1980s, a committee examining the infrastructure of the county concluded that improving the health facilities was one of the top priorities. Still, there wasn't an agreed-upon plan to make improvements, and there was certainly no plan for raising the capital. Even crude estimates suggested that approximately $25 to $45 million was needed in investments, depending on the degree to which we developed a primary care service to complement our preventive personal services. Additionally, public climate was not favorable to raising money; in recent years, several bond and sales tax referendums for other purposes had been defeated during special elections.

I believed that we should try to put the bond issue before the people of DeKalb County for a vote. For several reasons I believed that voters would support the idea even if it meant a small property tax increase. First, I was aware of the broad and positive contact that our services had with the residents of DeKalb County. People were hearing the positive message of prevention services from many different places. Also, DeKalb County was one of a handful of counties being tracked by a major weekly new magazine during the upcoming presidential campaign, and polls were regularly showing that health was among the top concerns of our constituents. In November 1992, DeKalb County residents would be voting not only for president, but also for a new chief executive officer, for the long-time incumbent was finishing his second term, the most permitted by law.

Conventional wisdom advised against such an effort. Special elections, which generally resulted in low voter turnouts, were thought to favor passage because supporters were more likely to come out and vote. Further, there was no particular reason that health facilities would be immune from growing antigovernment sentiment. DeKalb County taxpayers had been increasingly vocal about their dislike of the tax burden they bore in subsidizing Grady Memorial Hospital, which was operated by the Fulton-DeKalb Hospital Authority. Lastly, if the referendum failed, it would be several years before the issue could be raised again.

A unanimous vote of the county commission put the item on the ballot. The commissioners seem to have been decided by two things: the positive message inherent in the idea of prevention services and a video depicting our cramped facilities, which occupied small, aging buildings. Hearing and vision tests were being conducted in a closet at one health center, and at another, the confidentiality of young mothers was being compromised during counseling sessions because of lack of space; these problems shocked our elected officials. Additionally, the video was a dramatic substitute for the visits officials found hard to work into their busy schedules. Most commissioners said they thought placing the referendum on the ballot was a long shot but worth trying. None predicted that 62 percent of the voters would vote for its passage.

Three people stood out among the large group of remarkable people who worked for the passage of the referendum for improved health facilities: Mr. Fred Agel, our board chairman; Ms. Verna Barrett, our director of public relations, recruited out of retirement; and Mrs. Barbara Loar, recently retired director of the DeKalb Library System. These people knew the county and were tireless volunteers. They responded to the positive message we were trying to communicate. They appreciated being asked to participate, and they knew that our senior staff would help them any time, day or night.

We modeled our community assessment activity on that recommended by the Assessment Protocol for Excellence in Public Health (APEX/PH) protocol, which the National Association of County and City Health Officials recommends. Our community committee was called the Status of Health (SOH) committee. Under the leadership of its chairman, Robert Brown, an architect, and with support from the board of health and from Grady Memorial Hospital, the SOH committee established a Small Grants Program that would fund prevention projects with amounts of no more than $5,000. Over the past three years, 136 community and neighborhood groups have received grants, averaging about $3,500 each, to undertake specific primary prevention activities.

The small grants have supported a wide variety of efforts. One neighborhood group organized a summer arts program that involved youth in producing plays about solutions to their problems. Another group, provocatively called Bosom Buddies, provided outreach within the Hispanic community to arrange for mammograms. Parents Against Crack provided tutorials and computer experience after school. Volunteers from a disability service agency surveyed high-rise apartments for the elderly for injury prevention opportunities and replaced worn rubber stoppers on walkers so that older folks would be more stable while walking and avoid dangerous falls. These very productive voluntary efforts have fostered a countywide appreciation for prevention services and have built a constituency for the agency.

REORGANIZATION AND TRANSFORMATION

With the success of each of these efforts—in particular, the success of the passage of the facilities bond referendum—our staff began to realize the value of our community constituency. At the same time, however, we were still internally structured in a way that focused on providing clinical services to the individual. Then, with the governor's support, the state legislature passed a law in February 1994 reforming the state mental health system. This law had two results: Responsibility for directing the mental health section was taken away from the local health director, and an agency separate from the Board of Health took responsibility for the program. Almost overnight our agency shrank from 1,000 to approximately 400 employees; moreover, our smaller agency focused solely on public health.

In a process lasting a little more than a year, from July 1994 to August 1995, we capitalized on this change, completely reorganizing the staff and programs of the Board of Health. This took a full 13 months because we formed nine workgroups to flesh out our general vision for a new structure and to plan the transition to make it a reality. Each group developed a mission and a workplan and reported their progress to a transition council comprised of the chairpersons of the workgroups.

The transformation continues. We now have major organizational units focused on policy development, information services, community health promotion, and environmental health. We have decentralized our clinical operations into five major health centers, each pursuing integrated, comprehensive, primary care preventive services, in partnership with a primary care partner who is linked with a managed care system.

Our experience over the past year in preparation for offering managed care in the metropolitan Atlanta area led me to describe our aspirations in a speech at the most recent American Public Health Association (APHA) meeting:

> Initially, we are working to bring about reform for the people we currently serve, and eventually for our total population. We hope it will be so attractive that change will flourish and will be emulated and joined by the private sector. There are two marriages in this vision. The first is between the Board of Health, with its supportive home visits, outreach, and clinical preventive services, and the Grady Health System, with its primary medical care, and medical specialty and hospital services. We are also exploring a similar partnership with Oakhurst Community Health Center. We are developing relationships with commercial managed care entities to augment our outreach services. The central core of this marriage is the integrated comprehensive primary care at each of our new health centers.
>
> The second marriage is between this circle of personal services and the foundation of public health core functions of health information (which include information systems, surveillance, and epidemiology), environmental health, and community health promotion.
>
> We call this a "distinctive competency" because we believe that it exists nowhere else in the Atlanta managed care market. It has three components:
>
> 1. integrated comprehensive primary care
> 2. a foundation of broad population-based services
> 3. managed care plans and systems
>
> One concrete example may illustrate what we mean: A child is brought to a health center for a routine health screening. Our nursing staff discovers that the child has elevated levels of lead in his blood. Our primary care provider begins evaluation of the need for immediate treatment. The Health Information Services Unit generates a statistical analysis of blood levels of lead in patients in the area. Environmental health professionals begin an assessment of exposure in the home, daycare center or school, and other locations. Community health promotion staff organize community groups to develop a lead-exposure

control program. Our outreach staff begins home visits as part of follow-up with the family, and other potentially exposed children are brought in to be evaluated in a clinical setting. No other entity can bring all these resources to bear on such a problem. Herein lies our distinctive competency.

We are not there yet by any means. We and our partners are facing the challenges that all face in developing constructive partnerships with new partners, managed care networks, and insurance plans. These challenges include mundane issues such as insufficient experience with cost-accounting and marketing; differing definitions of words like "community," "population," and "integration"; unfair fee splitting; turf guarding; and inadequate information systems. There are also all the usual problems that occur when entities try to move into a collaborative relationship; they include clashes of organization cultures, preoccupation with governance, hardening of our various categories, overpromising, secrecy, and gamesmanship. But we are still optimistic. We are optimistic because we have an energizing vision.

LESSONS LEARNED

What lessons did I learn? What would I do differently? What has worked and why? My biggest regret is that I did not spend more time on developing the understanding and commitment of our employees as we were reshaping our community relationship.

Importance of Internal Community

In fact, I should have put into practice with our internal community more of the same principles we used externally. We attempted some things, such as having brown bag lunches and training staff volunteers to work with the SOH projects. (The brown bag lunches were very successful for the first six to nine months, but then interest tended to wane.) We trained staff to do specific tasks such as making presentations or conducting surveys for the SOH program but failed to provide the overall context and rationale for how this effort was aligned with the new vision. When all was said and done, our internal constituency development was incomplete, and only recently, with the new reorganization, have more people become aligned with the vision. This has been due, in large part, to our following the advice that we received from Joyce Essien and Jane Nelson after they completed an in-depth survey of our staff.

Developing an internal constituency requires more in quality and quantity than I recognized in our first efforts. The interviews of our staff by Drs. Essien and

Nelson revealed an ambivalence in regard to the concept of community owner-ship, a limited skill base in group facilitation, a continued focus on personal care, and an incomplete dissemination of information about our essential public health activities. Qualitatively, we had, and still have, a lot of work to do to transmit the basic concepts and to develop ownership for the ideas. But I also suspect that I missed the quantitative aspects of internal constituency development. Employees need to be given large numbers of opportunities to have a dialogue about issues. Leaders and senior people, including myself, tend to underestimate the sheer vol-ume of communication that is necessary for organizational transformation.

An important aspect of good local public health practice is maintaining relation-ships with elected officials. Recognizing the contributions of elected officials tends to build more sustained institutional support for public health. But it must be remembered that the job of the chief executive officer of a local public health agency is distinctly different from that of the chief executive officer of a private business. Local public health leaders are entrusted with power and influence be-cause, in a democracy, the public has entrusted that role to their elected officials. Elected officials transfer that trust to the directors of public health agencies. In Georgia, the transfer occurs because a state statute establishes the local boards of health, that is, in recognition of the statute, local county commissioners appoint the members of the Board of Health who govern my activities and the actions of agency staff. Civic lessons aside, there is something impressive about these rela-tionships. Finding ways to recognize elected officials and the people they appoint contributes to the civility and integrity of a community.

Contributions of Elected Officials

Collins led the fight for the Clean Indoor Air Ordinance. We mainly provided technical and organizational support. While we initially didn't have a highly vis-ible champion for the facility bond referendum among the elected officials, sev-eral important officials supported us. Our reorganization required the conscien-tious oversight of our board. Perhaps it is at the local level of politics that this is a most important lesson to learn. The need to make immediate decisions and to recognize the link between those decisions and their specific consequences re-quires a respect for the political process. This is not to say that a public health director should inject himself or herself into local politics in a partisan manner. To do so would result in a loss of legitimate power and positive influence on behalf of the public's health.

If I were to do it all over again, I would invest more in training staff in the techniques and strategies that help mobilize communities to action. I would have reorganized sooner and introduced earlier and in a more formal way, the principles of continuous improvement of quality public health services. What modest success we've had is based on maintaining a reasonably clear idea about where we were headed, then attracting others to that vision, and viewing our public health efforts as a mission. We found that scanning the external and internal environment is essential, as is using formal and informal means of communication. It is also useful to seek out conflict, not to submerge it, to clarify issues, and to listen carefully. Additionally, it helps to have a sense of humor and to count on making mistakes. A leader must be prepared to leave familiar turf and explore unknown communities and groups. A leader must also enjoy taking some risks. Experience has taught me that none of this would work if I had been unable to attract a team committed to the same ideals, or if I lacked faith in the strength and wisdom of people who live in our county.

I view our recent reorganization as the beginning of an internal transformation of our public health services. We will change even more as new opportunities arise. To be a part of this transformed relationship to our community is gratifying, and to begin to educate and to develop the skills of our staff is exhilarating.

CHAPTER 8

The Pope, Hot Pavement, and Public Health

Fernando A. Guerra

Serendipity is defined as the faculty for making fortunate and unexpected discoveries by accident. I suspect it plays a larger role in human affairs than most of us would care to acknowledge. I am convinced, however, that this phenomenon is not a completely random or chance occurrence. It depends in part on a person's experience, mind-set, and willingness to be open toward and accepting of the opportunities each day brings us for making new observations. I believe serendipity not only takes place but can be cultivated, and that reorganizing this quality will promote a better understanding of how leadership develops.

As I recollect my first days and weeks upon assuming the position of Director of Health for the City of San Antonio and Bexar County, I realize that I benefited from two serendipitous occurrences that subsequently shaped and formed much of my administration. The first—Pope John Paul's visit to San Antonio—was a unique experience that thrust me and my "new" department into the forefront of a major community celebration and national media event. The pope's visit served to bring home the many challenges facing any public health administrator in a large urban environment. The second example, an experience that led to the reassessment of our childhood immunization policies and procedures and eventually resulted in the refinement and expansion of our computerized immunization registry, will be described in some detail in the body of this article.

THE EARLY YEARS

My introduction to public health was an auspicious one, totally unexpected and unplanned. A pediatrician active in a small group practice, with credentials in public health, I was at the time of my career change the part-time director of a community and migrant worker health center. One August evening, I received a phone call from an assistant city manager inviting me to a breakfast meeting the following morning; at this meeting I was asked to consider appointment as interim Director of Health for the San Antonio Metropolitan Health District (SAMHD). The previous director had resigned on short notice, and amid some contention, leaving the city without a public health leader while facing national attention as the host of a papal visit that would take place in less than four weeks.

City officials were anxious that the necessary public health and public safety assurances might not be in place to handle the anticipated half-million visitors. San Antonio's summer climate, heat and humidity, poses special challenges in caring for large gatherings of people, especially in an outdoor environment. Adequate shelter from the heat, potable water, portable toilets, first aid supplies, and an effective triage system for medical care were at the top of the list for attention. Political pressures and expectations for a smooth and uneventful celebration were felt by all, and so by necessity my learning curve had to be short and steep. I had to assess the capabilities of my new department in very short order as well as develop effective linkages with other municipal services that were equally important support roles.

In the end, all of the hectic preparations, the intense planning, and the meticulous coordination paid off. The visit by Pope John Paul II and 450,000 other guests was a great success, but more important from my perspective was that our carefully constructed public health infrastructure had held up under pressure. More than 4,000 people received medical care by triage and 60 persons with more serious conditions were transported to hospitals by either ambulance or helicopter.

There were no major crises, only the usual medical emergencies and interventions that would be expected in such a large gathering were observed. Much of the credit for this record must be assigned to the staff I inherited on such short notice. Their ability to adapt to new and changing circumstances and perform at high levels of efficiency under stressful conditions is to their great credit. For me personally, it brought home the unique role public health can play in a community and gave new meaning to the term "population-based health care." It also represented an opportunity to more clearly formulate some thoughts on my own professional work and career direction. I began by examining options and opportunities afforded by public health to affect basic changes in a community, including improving health outcomes and raising awareness about wellness and healthy lifestyles. I came to appreciate the fact that the role of the public health authority gives one a very special podium, with unique access to the public. With that access goes the responsibility for its creative and responsible use to advance programs and priorities that most benefit the community's health and well being.

What started as an interim appointment to help the city through a difficult few weeks turned into a long-term commitment. I often reflect that whatever success I might have enjoyed during those early, challenging, and at times chaotic days was due to, rather than in spite of, the fact that I was in many ways unprepared for this adventure. I had neither an agenda nor preconceptions to burden me. I was determined, however, to seize whatever opportunities presented themselves and to be observant, flexible, and open. There is more than a little truth in the old adage, "Chance favors the prepared mind."

Some observations are so vivid and strong that they imprint themselves on my memory with a special clarity. During the middle of August in 1987, shortly after I was appointed the city's Director of Health and preparing for the papal visit, I had begun a series of introductory visits to our clinics to meet staff. The day I began the visits was as hot and humid as only a South Texas day can be. I had been in my new position only a few weeks and was visiting one of our community clinics in one of our poorer neighborhoods on the city's east side.

I intended to introduce myself to the staff and tour the facility, but as I parked my car I observed a woman cross the parking lot with four small children in tow. Several of the children were barefoot and hopping and skipping to escape touching the hot pavement. We entered the clinic at about the same time, and I observed her approach one of the nurses on duty to ask whether she could have her children immunized as school would be opening soon. The nurse was polite and attentive, but she informed the woman that the clinic did not offer immunizations on that particular day and that she would have to come back at a certain day and time. That short exchange, which turned out to be all too routine, came to symbolize in my mind a public health system that did not always serve the public as well as it should.

It was clear to me that this event presented me with a small window of opportunity that should be put to good use. Here was a mother who, with some effort and discomfort to herself and her children, had sought us out, but we could not accommodate her. It was obvious to me that, in this instance at least, public health had failed in its responsibility. Having made this observation, I concluded that perhaps what happened was an indication that other observations should be made during my initial days on the job; that would allow me to assess other aspects of our service delivery system and determine how "user friendly" my new department was.

Visits to other clinics in the days following brought to light other practices and patterns that, to the eyes of this newcomer, appeared questionable and counterproductive to the spirit and the mission of public health. I observed that nurses in our well-child and prenatal services clinics did not do immunizations. A division of labor designed to foster efficiency and develop expertise was in effect undermining the delivery of an essential and critical service. I saw that clinics were being shut down early to allow staff to catch up on paperwork or to accommodate in-service training programs. I noticed that our vital statistics division regularly closed its doors a half hour before the rest of our offices, routinely frustrating customers arriving and expecting service. It was clear that we had too many missed opportunities.

In looking at the larger picture, it is important to understand that I had inherited a public health bureaucracy comfortably ensconced within a larger city government bureaucracy. While public service, in all of its guises, is a noble calling, it can sometimes perpetuate an institutional mind-set that insulates people and discourages creativity and innovation. In that kind of a working environment, managers are not exposed to the same competitive forces that drive private sector enterprises. Issues of customer service, market research, quality assurance, and new product development are typically not high-priority concerns.

Not surprisingly, effecting change in such a climate is a slow and often frustrating process. The missed opportunities I identified were gradually being addressed, but often grudgingly. It was an evolutionary rather than a revolutionary change process. I came to recognize that my efforts to introduce change were not being resisted because of any principled opposition but rather more often by staff's simple business-as-usual attitude. This attitude existed at all levels, from senior administrative personnel assigned to the director's office to clinic staff assigned in the community to cashiers and receptionists.

I recognize now that perhaps the greatest single challenge facing a public health administrator in such an environment is how to redirect and reenergize staff with a new vision of public health as a public service. In some cases it calls for recruiting new staff and assuring that they have bought into this proactive value system. In more serious instances, staff might have to be removed, replaced, or reassigned. Over time, however, I was pleased to note steady progress in our efforts to instill a new pride in being identified with Metro Health—San Antonio's Public Health Team.

These first weeks constituted my introduction to the real world of public health, as opposed to the textbook model. Over time, I consciously tried to seek out opportunities to expand these kinds of observations to see where they would lead. I found that many systems in place were counterproductive, even counterintuitive as in the case of childhood immunizations. My sense was that public health was too often not energized or dynamic. In some instances, it lacked even responsiveness and accountability. In many cases we were satisfied with getting by rather than being on the cutting edge.

This initial impression, I now realize, was reflective of the prevailing state of public health in many communities across the nation. Public health had enjoyed an extended period where major accomplishments and successes were almost routinely expected and carried us all along. This golden age was being followed by one of apathy, in which our formerly proactive posture was being replaced by acceptance and complacency. I am pleased to note that the pendulum has swung back in recent years, and that we are now seeing a new re-energized, more focused, and creative public health movement taking center stage once again.

Immunizations have been and are an integral part of our core services. These initial emerging experiences led me to a fuller, more detailed examination of this program and its operating policies and procedures. A review of our community statistics revealed that there was considerable room for improvement in our performance. There were barriers we ourselves were erecting, albeit unconsciously in most cases. Gradually, I was able to identify and dismantle several of these real or perceived barriers. Clinic hours, locations, and scheduling were revamped with priority given to client convenience. Staff were cross-trained and encouraged to aggressively pursue opportunities to expand services. The success and enthusiasm engendered by these experiments resulted in an immunization program model that attracted national attention. It also laid the foundation and created the climate that encouraged us to move childhood immunizations into the computer era and the modern information age. We are still in the initial stages of that journey, and the next section of this article will recount the highlights of that adventure.

THE EVOLUTION OF A SYSTEM

Just as an effective public health presence provides the essential foundation and infrastructure for a community's varied health care enterprises, so does a childhood immunization program serve as a keystone in any public health strategy. Long recognized as one of the most cost-efficient prevention initiatives available to health care professionals, childhood immunization enjoys growing support and awareness from the public at large as well as from a broad range of policy makers at all levels of government. This is largely the result of active education and social marketing campaigns conducted in communities across the nation, which have helped introduce many new, safe, and effective vaccines.

On a practical and political level, the design and development of such initiatives reveal much about the role of the institution of public health within a community's overall health care delivery system. This is even truer today, in a climate of diminishing resources, shifting roles and responsibilities, and competition for market share. In addition to describing my introduction to public health, this article represents an effort to capture the contribution that reflects San Antonio's experience with the development and implementation of a computerized tracking system for its childhood immunization program. The current system, which is continually evolving, allows for accurate tracking, monitoring, and outreach activities essential for maintaining maximum compliance with the recommended immunization schedules and standards as well as the identification and targeting of underserved and underimmunized populations. Its effectiveness in surveillance, and as a management tool in inventory control, has also been well documented.

Like so many innovations that were destined to have impact but resulted in unintended consequences, the introduction of modern computer-based data collection technology to San Antonio's immunization program had modest origins. Even in the 1970s, when this particular system development began, the SAMHD had made its presence known as the public health agency serving the neediest neighborhoods. Then, as is the case today, there was an ongoing struggle to maintain a network of community-based health care services to provide the public with a safety net for at-risk populations. While the term "information age" was not in use at the time, there was a growing awareness among health professionals that the old methods of documenting care, namely file cabinets overflowing with medical records and government forms, were becoming increasingly unmanageable.

The very success of the SAMHD's various childhood immunization initiatives compounded this dilemma. Our network of community-based neighborhood clinics delivered not only immunization services but also a broad range of maternal and child health services and a variety of prevention, early intervention, and health education programs. SAMHD found itself drawn into an ever more prominent leadership role over time, not only as an advocate of improved childhood immunization compliance, but also as the lead agency in delivering the service to the community. Our client base, as experience was teaching us, was often very mobile. In many cases the children in these families had multiple caregivers attending to their medical needs across public and private sectors. With Spanish as the primary, and in some cases the only, language of a large segment of our clientele, accurate communication became a major concern. Multiple records were being created at different clinic sites, frequently under different names. This became an administrative nightmare even before it surfaced as a clinical management issue or a public health problem interfering with assessment, monitoring, or outreach planning.

Growing awareness of the benefits of computerized databases in improving the accuracy, comprehensiveness, and accessibility of client information caused SAMHD to open an exploratory dialogue with San Antonio's Information Services Department. This division was charged with the comprehensive task of defining citywide and interdepartmental strategies to bring the programs and services of city government into the information age. Modest steps were initiated to standardize data collection and entry from paper records shipped to the central administrative offices from remote clinic sites. As the information was gathered, it was entered into the city's mainframe computer. For the first time, this created a common database that allowed for review and a limited analysis of geographic coverage and rates of compliance for the population served through the department's clinics. These beginning steps were of most interest to those charged with policy planning, budget development, and resource allocation. The data represented a relatively crude indication of activity driven by local clinic input of their paper files, but unfortunately there was little opportunity for timely feedback to the local service delivery site and the clinicians staffing them.

Building on the original database that centralized information in the city's mainframe computer, a revised and enhanced system was developed with active support and encouragement from the Centers for Disease Control and Prevention (CDC) and the city's Information System Department (ISD). A new program was created for vaccine inventory, storage, and distribution to health department clinics, physicians, and other providers in the system. Another modification was subsequently added for improved tracking capability. Quarterly reminders were sent out to every child in the system who was 90 days delinquent in reporting his or her immunization status. Finally, a separate microfiche system was added to complement the system and was made available to over 150 providers, 16 school districts, and the hospital district to verify students' vaccination status.

At the start of the 1980s, the system was little more than a static registry, but as the decade closed out, a sophisticated tracking system was taking shape that showed real promise as a valuable tool for improving San Antonio's record for compliance with recommended immunization schedules. The 1980s were characterized by continual refinements and revisions to the database and the software supporting it. There was modification to the vaccine distribution system, further improvement in client tracking, and the creation of more efficient and user friendly forms of automation. For those missing appointments, reminder notices were routinely sent out on a monthly basis, rather than every quarter as had been the case previously. Client noncompliance after two reminder notes triggered phone contacts or home visits by public health nurses.

The 1990s have seen strong and consistent support from both the public and private sectors in recognition of this pioneering work. The CDC again provided additional resources for hardware acquisition, software upgrades, and more sophisticated vaccine reporting procedures. The birth record became a central feature and a point of entry into this new system. All records were transferred to a special database, and thereafter every birth record was entered into the registry and the immunization tracking system, but only after the child had become part of the SAMHD immunization program by visiting one of its clinics or affiliated public or private sector providers. Most important, these new resources have allowed for the regular inclusion of more than 22,000 newborns from the annual registry to the tracking system. The infants are added to the database with an actual record, which in most instances includes the date of the first dose of hepatitis B. This process has allowed providers to send their immunization information to the health department that became, de facto, the immunization record keeper of almost two-thirds of the population of children up to 18 years of age.

The Robert Wood Johnson Foundation funded a demonstration project to expand the community-based network and enhance our tracking system. Computers were added to all health department clinics and to a group of 20 private providers who became part of the on-line system, accessing and simultaneously updating the health department's records. Shortly thereafter, the Merck, Sharp and Dohme Company entered into a partnership with SAMHD to demonstrate immunization services in a children's hospital emergency department. A total of three hospitals were eventually included and as part of the demonstration were also connected to the immunization services database and tracking system in the emergency department, pediatric ward, outpatient clinic, and newborn nursery. In 1993, another revision allowed for the introduction of special coding and identifiers to track the immunization status of children on public assistance.

As we assess the current status and future direction of our Immunization Tracking System in 1996, and anticipate its future growth and development, a number of accomplishments should be noted. First, we need to appreciate that the SAMHD annually records over 385,000 immunizations. A network of 13 decentralized neighborhood clinics with flexible hours, walk-in services, and weekend coverage throughout the city provide these immunizations. Immunizations are also provided through our maternal and child health services; Early and Periodic Screening, Diagnosis and Treatment; family planning; and 13 Women's, Infants' and Children's Program sites. The project also monitors all school and childcare facilities for immunization compliance as well as providing special clinics for these groups. Vaccine is distributed to more than 372 private providers who administer over 195,000 doses of public vaccine and maintain highly accurate records of doses administered and to whom. The signed consent forms serve to update the immunization information for each client.

Currently, the computerized system holds more than 650,000 client files with multiple immunization records. It serves as the principal database for immunization records, compliance analysis, the reminder/delinquent notification system, and the adverse event register, and it also serves as the basis of a vaccine accountability system. This database is increasing by almost 24,000 new births each year. The system serves both providers and clients, both of whom can access the system for record verification and copies. A recall postcard is generated on a quarterly basis for anyone under five years of age who has not returned within 30 days of their due date. These are followed up by our staff to assure compliance. The system at any given moment can provide random sampling of immunization compliance by age, geographic area, or by public and private provider. Through the different assessments done from birth record cohorts, we have estimated that 98 percent of all children under 2½ years of age born in Bexar County have a record in our system.

There are several goals addressed by the immunization tracking system as it is currently configured. The first is basically an issue of client compliance and service management. We strive to record and track the immunization given to each child to ensure that each child receives the correct vaccine on schedule, and in appropriate dosage; we wish to minimize either overimmunization or underimmunization due to misplaced or incomplete records by the parent or guardian. New bar coding technology is allowing us to enhance our efficiency in this area. Each client will be assigned a unique bar code that represents a personal identification number. Registering a client will require scanning the bar code of the immunization record to pull up the demographic and immunization history of the client. Vaccines to be administered will be scanned in from a universal vaccine bar code sheet. The consent form for the current visit is then printed, and an updated immunization record is given to each client at each visit. Manufacturer and lot number of the day will automatically be inserted for each vaccine at the time of registration. This latter feature is especially important since it allows us to react promptly to any adverse reactions reported and link the client with a specific vaccine lot should a follow-up or recall be indicated.

State-of-the-art auto-dialer technology is just now being incorporated into our system. This will allow providers and school nurses to call in and receive the latest immunization record of anyone on the tracking system. It will also allow the public to call and receive the immunization schedule or the immunization needed based on a given birth date. General information about clinic locations, hours, and basic directions can also be programmed into the system. Nightly, the auto-dialer will call parents whose children are behind on their immunizations and remind them to receive their immunizations. They will be given the location of a clinic nearest to them and the system will even allow the parent to leave a message for the Health District Immunization staff should they so desire.

Our tracking system, unlike those in many other communities, incorporated inventory control early on in its development. It tracks all inventory received from the manufacturer and also documents which provider receives the vaccine. Data entry staff at the main clinic adjust the inventory for the clinic on a nightly basis. Neighborhood clinics and providers in our network mail in the consent forms at the end of each month so the inventory for those clinics is adjusted on a monthly basis. The next logical step to improve and expand the tracking system will be to incorporate bar coding into the inventory system. This will greatly enhance the efficiency of control and distribution functions.

We are at a critical juncture in strategic planning and policy development as we determine the way our present system will meet the needs of the 21st century. How the immunization tracking system can be linked to other health district programs, other city department databases, and alternative information system technologies sponsored by state and federal agencies will be the principal challenge for the immediate future.

In the Institute of Medicine's seminal work *The Future of Public Health*, public health is defined as "fulfilling society's interest in assuring conditions in which people can be healthy."[1] Those of us who have enjoyed the great honor of serving in this cause know that it has a strong history, a clear vision, and a challenging agenda. My early days in public health were played out against a background of rapid and profound change in our field, a paradigm in the field that persists to the present day. In spite of this, by choice or by serendipity, it has provided many enriching and gratifying experiences to me personally. In turn, my experiences have reinforced my sense of the need to be open, alert, flexible, and responsive to the unique opportunities offered to us by life's experiences. Can that chance encounter with a mother and her children in the parking lot so many years ago be credited with bringing about our present day high-tech tracking system? Perhaps not, but I remain convinced that it opened a window somewhere. One never knows what will be "blowing in the wind [. . . of opportunity]."

REFERENCE

1. Institute of Medicine. *The Future of Public Health*. Washington, D.C.: National Academy Press, 1988.

PART IV

Public Health Programming

CHAPTER 9

Building Collaborative Bridges Between Public Health and Health Care Delivery: Leadership Strategies for New Partnerships

Susan J. Klein

When New York City experienced a resurgence of tuberculosis (TB) in the 1980s, we found that public health and health care resources were insufficient to assure effective public health disease prevention and adequate care of the many individuals in New York City with TB. Nonadherence to prescribed antituberculosis treatment regimens can contribute to further the spread of TB in the community, development of multidrug-resistant TB, escalation of health care costs related to hospitalizations and rehospitalizations, and increased morbidity and mortality. Inadequate treatment contributed to an increase in the proportion of drug-resistant cases, and we experienced outbreaks of multidrug-resistant TB in several New York City hospitals.

There were inadequate public health resources in New York City to offer directly observed therapy to all individuals who could benefit from it. The health care delivery system was unprepared to provide proper care and treatment for the large number of individuals with TB. Yet addressing the burgeoning epidemic required the skills, dedication, and commitment of both sectors.

Within the New York State Department of Health (NYSDOH), I was part of a small group of individuals who identified several aspects of the TB epidemic re-

The author thanks Dr. Lloyd F. Novick, Onondaga County Health Department; Dr. Guthrie S. Birkhead and Wendy Shotsky, New York State Department of Health; Richard Goldberg, Mount Sinai Medical Center of New York City; and Gail Cairns, New York City Department of Health, for their review of the manuscript. This article is dedicated to the staff who worked with me and to colleagues from other organizations whose personal and professional contributions made this extraordinary experience possible.

99

quiring immediate policy attention from the very highest levels of New York State government. A major issue was nonadherence to treatment, which we presented to the New York State legislature in 1990–1991.

I will never forget walking with my colleagues Drs. George DiFerdinando, Dale Morse, and Lloyd Novick through the quarter-mile underground passageway that linked our building in Albany to the legislative office building. On the way to meet with the chairman of the New York State Assembly Health Committee, we attached rough cost estimates to each of a series of 10 "bullets," each of which was a policy recommendation to stem the TB epidemic. The result was authorization by the New York State legislature and the governor to proceed with the development of enhanced programs to help assure completion of TB treatment, using Medicaid as a funding mechanism.

WHY WAS LEADERSHIP NEEDED? WHY ME?

Development of an appropriate and effective intervention required both immediate attention and leadership; existing systems were not working, and the public's health was directly threatened. The severity of the epidemic necessitated the timely development of an intervention that would have to span the public health and health care sectors to be effective. A creative approach, representing a departure from current practice, was required. There were multiple stakeholders to be contacted and mobilized, including the New York City Department of Health (NYCDOH), which received separate funds for TB prevention and which was also in the process of formulating its own response to the epidemic. The involvement of multiple stakeholders would have to be coordinated.

I was requested by the executive deputy director of the Office of Public Health to become directly involved in the development of an appropriate response that entailed integrating TB directly observed therapy (DOT) into the activities of already existing health care providers in New York City. (DOT is a method of ensuring patient adherence to the TB treatment regimen. It entails observation of the patient ingesting antituberculosis medications by a public health care provider or other trained person.) The objective was to revise the existing health care system to provide adequate capacity for provision of DOT. Successfully approaching this problem required an intervention consonant with the objectives and operations of a diverse group of community providers.

Addressing nonadherence to treatment regimens required a multidisciplinary approach. Not only would public health officials from the state and city need to cooperate in a strategic fashion but so would doctors, nurses, social workers, infection control practitioners, laboratorians, administrators, and outreach workers.

I was not part of the already existing specific TB prevention and control infrastructures of either the state or the city, yet I possessed organizational standing by virtue of my role as associate director of the Division of Epidemiology, which houses the state's Bureau of Tuberculosis Control. At the time, I was also acting director of the division. I had substantial experience in public health planning, community coalition development, and public health capacity building, as well as knowledge of administrative and financial mechanisms. I was regarded as someone who could be relied on to ensure that the myriad details inherent in accomplishing a goal would not be overlooked.

THE ENVIRONMENTAL SCAN: STAKEHOLDERS AND CONFLICTING AGENDAS ABOUNDED

My review of the internal and external environments quickly confirmed many potential barriers to success. For example, the New York City health care system was notorious for being pluralistic and discordant. It was characterized by competition and driven by local politics. Within the city, the relationship between the municipal hospital system and the public health system was strained; turf issues abounded. I found little apparent communication or cooperation around issues of TB prevention in the early 1990s. Competition between municipal and voluntary hospitals in New York City for reimbursement and other resources was fierce. Municipal hospitals had historically served large numbers of hard-to-reach individuals lacking health insurance, including many with TB, without the requisite resources. Voluntary hospitals historically had access to the paying patients and greater resources; yet they, too, were unprepared for the growing numbers of TB patients coming to them for care.

The relationship between the state and city health departments was tense. The NYSDOH had statewide responsibility for TB control, but the NYCDOH had preceded NYSDOH historically and therefore had independent authority under many sections of the state public health law. Both health departments received public health funding directly from the Centers for Disease Control and Prevention (CDC). Despite the severity of the epidemic, in 1991 the state and the city were not collaborating on many issues key to tuberculosis control.

There were numerous administrative impediments and obstacles. Amendment of the state plan for Medicaid was required to reimburse providers for TB DOT; this needed approval from the Health Care Financing Administration (HCFA). There were legal issues to be resolved, such as scope of practice. And, since not everyone was eligible for or enrolled in Medicaid, to offer TB DOT in a widespread manner would require the development of other financial resources and reimbursement streams.

Principal stakeholders noted above were at odds and were even competitive. Mistrust between the various governmental agencies and among the hospitals flourished, and cooperation between public health agencies and health care organizations was minimal. Other organizations serving individuals with TB and the patients themselves were additional stakeholders. More often than not, these other organizations (primarily clinics, social service providers, housing providers, community-based organizations, and human immunodeficiency virus/acquired immunodeficiency syndrome [HIV/AIDS] care and service providers) were leery of TB control efforts, yet their cooperation was critical.

In addition, the patients themselves had to accept the concept of TB DOT. It was not a foregone conclusion that people would accept TB DOT, since it could be perceived as a regulatory control and an invasion of privacy. Many individuals have an inherent mistrust of governmental programs, and others contend that the epidemic is the fault of those suffering with the disease. Our experience providing care and services to people with HIV/AIDS in New York City highlighted and magnified these dynamics.

IMPLEMENTATION PLANNING

Planning to implement the program began in August 1991. Meetings held between the NYSDOH and the New York State Department of Social Services (NYSDSS) resulted in an action plan based on specific strategies, which included the use of existing providers, Medicaid payment to providers for TB DOT services via a weekly fee, a flexible design to foster innovation on the part of providers to meet patient needs, and a team approach to program development. Numerous meetings with providers and representatives of state and city agencies, community-based organizations, social service providers, and academic institutions were necessary to work out the program in detail so that the overall program plan would have integrity, be realistic and, most important, enable individuals to complete their antituberculosis treatment regimens.

I had limited preexisting working relations with the traditional health care providers in New York City. Early meetings with providers to discuss our plans were chaired by the executive deputy director of the NYSDOH Office of Health Systems Management. This person was particularly successful in getting provider representatives to the table. However, meetings were contentious concerning labor and scope of practice issues, actual expectations for the public health activities we were asking health care providers to undertake, reimbursement, legal issues, and the interface between health care delivery and public health. These first meetings were called by the arm of the department that regulates and imposes penalties on the provider community, contributing to the initial confrontational dynamic. Often there would be 60 or more people in attendance from competing organizations with conflicting goals, ostensibly there for a working meeting.

Eventually, I was able to draft the actual scope of service for TB DOT based upon a consensus process of persons from various disciplines representing approximately 40 acute care facilities and their trade organizations, the state and city health departments, experts in health economics and reimbursement, and representatives of the NYSDSS. (In New York State, the NYSDSS was responsible for administration of the Medicaid program.)

What Were the Risks?

The venture of implementing provider-based DOT entailed multiple elements of risk. The sheer scale of this initiative and its urgent nature were striking. I itemized numerous technical and administrative uncertainties, and the list was overwhelming. Mobilizing public and voluntary health care providers to perform TB DOT as a public health function had never before been attempted on such a large scale.

This initiative involved collaboration among individuals, agencies, and organizations with long histories of not cooperating. I needed to foster a collaboration in an environment where this was the exception and not the rule. If the potential partners did not participate, I would not be able to deliver a cohesive program. Even more uncertain was whether this model would be successful in assisting individuals to complete their antituberculosis treatment. Patients, providers, the NYCDOH, and referring facilities had to agree to work together. I was not certain that individuals with TB would ever accept directly observed therapy, as it can be perceived as intrusive.

The incidence and prevalence of TB can be measured. Individuals receiving DOT can be, and eventually were, counted. There are quantifiable benchmarks that can be used to measure progress and success in the implementation at such a program. There was the worry that if this program worked, the numbers of infected patients and revenue for participating providers would go down. How could I motivate providers to engage in this venture when success would mean that the grants and reimbursement supporting the staff providing DOT would someday disappear?

Inadequate treatment is worse than none at all. A poorly designed program could contribute to, rather than stem, the epidemic. I possessed only a very basic understanding of the nature of TB and the various treatment modalities. I needed staff, access to internal expertise, help from NYCDOH, and the cooperation of individuals within provider settings to supplement my knowledge and skills. The stress I experienced while taking on the risky nature of this initiative was compounded by the fact that it was also highly visible. Sustained strong support from the NYSDOH was also absolutely critical in the face of internal and external tensions.

What Were the Benefits?

I recognized that the successful development of the DOT initiative would require cooperation, communication, and collaboration across sectors. In essence, what I needed to develop was a team approach to program development, with the team transcending the NYSDOH. Once the initial broad stokes had been negotiated with state and city agencies and providers, responsibility for working out the details for full implementation fell to me. To overcome initial hostility, I adopted a strategy of engaging individuals at high, but not too high, levels within the provider facilities and state and city governments as part of a team of peers.

Team facilitation skills were used to begin to break down barriers and provide a shared vision and focus for our work. Such an approach would minimize risks; assure identification of all pertinent details by bringing diverse perspectives to bear on the needs and issues; promote active, involved commitment; and lend enhanced credibility to the work. I was convinced that the intervention would benefit greatly from the combined power of the expertise and credibility of all participants.

In addition, I envisioned that long-term benefits would accrue from a partnership developed around TB DOT. Individuals, contacts, and relationships that bridged public health and health care delivery would undoubtedly serve us well in the future in unexpected ways.

DEVELOPING THE TEAM, STRATEGIES, AND BENEFITS

I knew from my previous experience in community health planning and coalition development that several elements would be critical to developing a team that spanned sectors.

Clarity on Our Ultimate Goal and Mission

A very specific focus on completion of antituberculosis treatment regimens would enable timely integration of DOT into activities of providers throughout the five boroughs of New York City. We sought to ensure that TB DOT should be accessible and available to all individuals with TB, regardless of their insurance status or ability to pay.

We adopted a patient-centered approach to planning, a holistic model that captured other determinants of health (access to health care, housing, entitlement, nutrition, etc.) whenever possible, but always with the goal of TB treatment completion in mind.

This focus provided a solid foundation for team building and working through diverse and controversial issues. Always, when the going got rough, we would remind ourselves of our goal and mission. I have a vivid image of one member of the team who would repeatedly remind us to consider what this would mean from the point of view of the patient. She had very long fingers and would point while saying this. This gentle but poignant reminder would influence our discussions and highlight how we should proceed.

Early Involvement

Early program planning involvement of city-based hospital and clinic providers as well as New York City agencies facilitated team development. Well before we announced the program model and invited city providers to respond to our request for proposals to offer TB DOT, we engaged the city health department, the individual municipal hospitals and their parent organization (the NYC Health and Hospitals Corporation [NYCHHC]), voluntary hospitals and their trade organization (the Greater New York Hospital Association [GNYHA]), and others in review of the program model, discussion of the scope of services to be offered, and the proposed reimbursement methodology. Numerous iterations reflecting these organizations' input and recommendations formed the final solicitations for additional providers to supplement the DOT available through the NYCDOH.

Playing to the interests of other parties is one technique that promoted early involvement. Labor unions representing health care workers in New York are very powerful and influential. I stressed the value of DOT as a "worker protection" strategy. Similarly, discussions with HCFA about the cost-effectiveness of DOT well before our state plan amendment was submitted helped pave the way for quick approval. HCFA Region II staff often attended our provider meetings and seemed proud that this cutting-edge public health work was occurring in their region.

Early involvement of diverse parties sent an important message that the NYSDOH did not think it had all the answers and that it viewed others as equal partners in this venture. I used sign-in sheets from meetings to identify individuals and organizations with an interest in and potential for contributing. Subsequent contacts resulted in ongoing relationships with individuals, many of whom would eventually become pillars of the team.

Creation of a Peer Network

Individuals within the separate health care facilities that agreed to offer TB DOT would be central to its successful widespread implementation. These individuals knew, and would learn firsthand, the obstacles, barriers, and successful strategies associated with DOT. We in state and city government could provide a supportive context for the program model, but only those directly involved in carrying it out on a day-to-day basis would know what it took to initiate and sustain effective programs.

I needed to develop mutually supportive relationships between myself, my staff, and individuals from hospitals and clinics, and we did our best from within the department to empower them to succeed. Many became TB DOT program managers or oversaw TB DOT programs within their facilities. In particular, representatives from Bellevue Hospital Center, Beth Israel Medical Center, GNYHA, Montefiore Medical Center, Mount Sinai Medical Center, South Brooklyn Health Center, St. Clare's and St. Vincent's Hospital of New York were involved from the beginning and became close and trusted colleagues. Staff of the NYCDOH and NYCHHC also joined this inner circle, providing invaluable advice and assistance.

Provider objections involved issues such as the scope of practice, a sense of uncertainty as to what was expected, and availability of adequate resources. Once I explored their concerns, it was clear that these were well founded. I worked with the State Education Department (SED) Board for Nursing and the chief counsel of the SED to resolve anxieties about the involvement of nurses in what was first construed as the "dispensing" of medications, which is outside the scope of practice for nurses licensed in New York State. I developed new resources for start-up grants and program enhancement grants for the DOT. Increased access to antituberculosis medications was possible through programs for the uninsured HIV-positive patient and through the NYCDOH pharmacy. As we gained experience with TB DOT, the inadequacy of the initial program protocols became evident, and we moved to replace them with program standards.

I chaired meetings for TB DOT program managers, which were held in New York City, as we began to put this program into place. At first these meetings primarily consisted of presentations and updates by me and others from state agencies. I tried to facilitate dialogue between the program managers and representatives of the NYCDOH; eventually these meetings became forums for dynamic discussions of issues and for problem-solving. Program managers became resources for each other; more experienced and senior individuals became mentors for less experienced managers from other hospitals or clinics. The NYCDOH, NYCHHC, and GNYHA became actively involved with this new program, too.

The strength of this peer network and our shared focus on completion of treatment on the part of individual patients greatly facilitated interhospital referrals. With our ultimate goal in mind, revenue and patient census considerations took a back seat to assuring the optimal provider-patient match. Competition for patients was secondary to continuity of care and successful completion of treatment.

The state and city health departments had different goals. The state health department invested heavily in the new program model, and there was considerable pressure to demonstrate high enrollment in the new hospital- and clinic-based programs. The city health department sought to maintain responsibility and control of as many TB patients as possible, both for public health reasons and, I suspected, to capture the new reimbursement. At first, I approached the monthly state-city conference calls with anxiety and apprehension. Later I began to look forward to talking with my new friends and colleagues.

Many of us from the two health departments made professional and personal commitments to our shared goal, the completion of treatment. We did not let the difficult dynamics between our two agencies get in the way of our work. In fact, since many contended that what we were seeking to put into place could not be done, we were highly motivated to assure its success and beat the odds. A network of persons with "just enough" policy-level discretion and clout can accomplish quite a bit without raising issues to levels where intergovernmental turf and political posturing can get in the way. A workable process evolved over many months, and in the end, we were all proud of what we were able to achieve.

Use of Work Groups To Advance Completion of Tasks and Solidify Relationships

Our initiative to provide DOT was announced before many aspects of its implementation were fully developed. Still other vital program components only became apparent as implementation progressed. Many of these components were outside of my direct experience and involved working on the interface between public health and health care delivery.

I used a series of interdisciplinary work groups consisting of representatives of the state and city health departments and the provider community to develop training programs for outreach workers and discharge planners, to develop systems and procedures for referral and enrollment, and to develop data report forms. The growing network of persons involved in implementing provider-based TB DOT in New York City became a resource network for program development. I requested and began to receive real case studies of individual patients with TB. These challenged the program model and helped point the way to solutions. Once brought to completion, each project component served to further solidify our relationships. Shared credit for our accomplishments was very important.

The first example of an interdisciplinary work group was called the Discharge Planning Work Group. This group was urgently needed to set up systems and procedures for referral of persons with TB to DOT on discharge from New York City hospitals. A representative of the GNYHA offered to introduce a colleague and me to a few hospital directors of social work or discharge planning.

The second time I met with the hospital directors of social work or discharge planning, I invited representatives of the NYCDOH. NYCDOH was in the process of assigning public health advisers to each New York City hospital to conduct active surveillance and to assure continuity of care on hospital discharge. Reaction was fierce; the hospital discharge planners accused the NYCDOH of trying to do their jobs. Through detailed enumeration of activities and tasks, we successfully resolved misunderstandings between the two groups regarding the roles of hospital discharge planners and public health advisers from NYCDOH. We were able to maximize the contributions of both.

This Discharge Planning Work Group was extremely productive over a period of approximately three years. Its products included guidelines, a provider directory, brochures, a poster, in-services and training sessions, a continuity of care flow chart, and presentations to local and national audiences. For me, this particular work group remains a highlight of the project and of my experience in public health. It was the quintessential example of unexpectedly productive teamwork across sectors and disciplines.

Another such example was creation of the Continuous Quality Improvement Council. Its goal was to provide advice and expertise concerning development, assessment, improvement, and enhancement of the DOT program. I explored the availability of training for quality improvement and team facilitation available from the governor's Office of Employee Relations, and we attended three training sessions in New York City as a group. I found that this shared experience improved our ability to work together on many difficult issues. Our shared focus on making sure that individual patients completed treatment also enabled the ready identification of obstacles and barriers to continuity of care. One such challenge was assuring continuity of treatment for individuals on release from state and city prisons and jails, for inmates enrolled in work release programs, and for parolees.

When my New York City colleagues mentioned going to "the Island," I thought they were planning a vacation. I was wrong; they meant the Rikers Island Correctional Facility. My first trip there was unforgettable. "The Island" featured 10 prisons, a high-tech isolation facility for TB patients, and lots of ribbon razor. When a superintendent told me of a female prisoner who "arranged" to be incarcerated at Rikers Island for the birth of her fourth child because her other three had been born there, I gained a greater appreciation for the challenges raised by lack of access to health care in the community.

Our trips to the correctional facility solidified and motivated our work group, which met several times over the course of about 18 months. This group's work on assuring continuity of care for inmates released from Rikers Island became a prototype for similar work within the state prison system. The New York State Department of Correctional Services and the New York State Division of Parole began developing direct relations with community providers in order to implement a new system of care for inmates and parolees with TB.

These work groups developed individual identities and instilled a growing feeling of loyalty among members toward our work. Even when the Office of the Mayor of New York City initiated a citywide strategic planning process to prevent and control TB separate from any involvement with the state health department, representatives of individual municipal hospitals, the NYCDOH, and the NYCHHC assured that our work was acknowledged and facilitated, rather than endangered or subsumed, by the planning process.

Joint Promotion of Program Model

Given the complex nature of New York City's health care system, I needed to rely on others to be ombudsmen and ambassadors to inform and sell the community on this intervention and to add clout. Joint presentations planned and carried out by teams involving both state and city health departments, the NYCHHC, the GNYHA, the Discharge Planning Association of New York City, and individual providers were very effective. The NYCHHC and GNYHA were instrumental in generating a receptive and enthusiastic response on the part of their individual hospital constituents. We presented a strong and united front to the health care community and to other involved agencies. Sometimes I would lead, but often we determined that others from our team had greater credibility and influence with a particular audience. We each developed the ability to lead, facilitate, or follow as our needs and circumstances dictated. When necessary, we mobilized our individual constituencies to broaden the team.

We also went together to national meetings, such as the American Hospital Association and American Public Health Association, to jointly present our program model to the health care and public health communities. The Fall 1995 issue of the *Journal of Public Health Management and Practice* featured several articles about this work. This group of articles has received national attention and lends further credibility to our efforts. Moreover, helping each other complete these articles further strengthened the team. We supported each other's agencies and organizations to obtain grant funding for the DOT and other projects.

We developed a growing group of individuals from various state and city agencies and from the provider community who are concerned about the problem of homelessness and TB. Many of us participated individually in a series of hearings held at the New York Academy of Medicine and testified on behalf of the needs of the homeless individuals we were serving. Although for all practical purposes we made separate presentations, our comments and perspectives were carefully crafted to be mutually supportive of the issue at hand. We worked together and within our own organizations on policy and resource development around homelessness. There are now housing programs in New York City for homeless individuals with TB and those dually infected with HIV and TB, enabling them to complete their regimens under the DOT program.

LONG-TERM BENEFITS

The immediate benefits of this project included a remarkable increase in availability of accessibility to and enrollment in TB DOT in New York City. Treatment completion rates improved. Greater teamwork within individual agencies and hospitals, facilitated by this project, has promoted many aspects of TB control. Resources were enhanced as individuals and organizations decided to participate. As a result, the intervention had greater integrity and a strong impact on public health.

We also achieved acceptance of DOT as a standard practice in the treatment of TB by both hospital-based and private physicians and other providers in New

York City. This initiative focused new attention on nonadherence to completion of treatment as an important issue and fostered acceptance of DOT as an integral part of clinical practice. This additional outcome has profound significance for individual and public health in the city and state of New York. Recently DOT has been highlighted by the World Health Organization as vital to global control of TB.

The long-term benefits of the individual relationships built around our efforts to implement the DOT program have yet to accrue, yet we succeeded in bridging public health and health care delivery. I am confident that trust, ease in communication, and cooperation between members of our team will make future interactions around other issues easier.

Many health problems cut across the traditional boundaries of public health and health care delivery. It is highly likely that many of us will find ourselves working together in the future. On November 1, 1995, I became acting director of the Division of HIV Prevention within the NYSDOH AIDS Institute. In this capacity I have already interacted with several individuals whom I met in the course of developing the DOT initiative. We have a common theoretical base, a shared history, and personal rapport that we can build on in our efforts to prevent HIV infection.

All of us who were involved in the work described above obtained a deeper, firsthand understanding of the power of working together toward a goal of improved health. I carry this experience with me and continue to apply the lessons learned. Most important, individuals in the community and those returning to the community from correctional institutions receive better health care and public health services when the two sectors can begin to bridge the gap between them. As we move into an era of managed care, such collaborative bridges are increasingly recognized as vital to assure access, quality, and continuity of care.

CHAPTER 10

Public Health Leadership in Five Kentucky Appalachian Counties

Grace G. Eddison

Early in 1994, a request for proposals (RFP) was issued by the federal Rural Health Outreach Grant Program. The purpose of this RFP was to support new and innovative models for more effective integration and coordination of outreach and health care services delivery in rural areas. Applicants were required to develop consortium arrangements with two or more health care or social service organizations; each consortium member was required to contribute significantly to the goals of the project. As Commissioner of Health for the Gateway District Health Department, I became interested in this project as a means of addressing health, human, and educational service needs. (Such needs were identified by the Gateway Health Coalition, a collaborative body founded by the health department to facilitate coordination and collaboration among public and private providers and consumers in addressing public and private health issues in the five-county Gateway area.)

PERTINENT DEMOGRAPHICS

The Gateway District Health Department covers all five area development district counties—Bath, Menifee, Montgomery, Morgan, and Rowan. It is located within the Appalachian region of eastern Kentucky. These counties have the typical problems of the region: poverty, poor education, poor health status, and isolation. The geographic area encompasses 1,360 square miles; in 1994 the population was 70,413. In 1995, the percentage of persons below the poverty level in the Gateway area ranged from 21 percent in Montgomery County to 35 percent in Menifee County (designated as a shortage area for health manpower) to 37 percent in Morgan County: a total of 18,902 impoverished persons in the district. In 1990, the percentage of students graduating from high school ranged from 44.1 percent in Morgan to 46.0 percent in Menifee to 57.9 percent in Rowan. At that time,

Kentucky ranked next to last in the country in regard to students graduating from high school, and Gateway as a whole had an average of only 52 percent of students graduating from high school.

The five-year-average infant death rate from 1990 through 1994 for the Gateway area was 8.9 deaths per 1,000 births. In Menifee, the infant death rate was markedly increased, with an average at 15.4 deaths per 1,000 births. The 1992 "KIDS COUNT" score, a rating of children's home life published by the Kentucky Youth Advocates, indicated that the high rates resulted from a combination of six major factors: children in poverty, children in single-parent homes, infant mortality, birth with early prenatal care, teen births, and high school graduation. With a score of 37, the Gateway area was ranked inadequate (defined as less than 40). The two counties with inadequate scores were Menifee, with a score of 25 (ranked 119th in the state out of 120 counties), and Morgan, with a score of 29.

PRIOR HISTORY OF PUBLIC HEALTH LEADERSHIP IN GATEWAY

The Gateway Health Coalition was formed in 1986 after the receipt of a technical assistance grant award (no funds; the award consisted of three public health experts making one field trip each to the Gateway Health Department) from the American Public Health Association to begin the implementation of the Healthy Communities 2000: Model Standards. The coalition also received a limited grant award from the Robert Wood Johnson Foundation, which allowed the hiring of an executive director for the health coalition in its beginning years of development. At the time of our application to the Rural Health Outreach Grant Program, we had a coalition membership of 800 individuals representing a wide variety of health and human service agencies, schools, universities, law enforcement, the judicial system, local and state government, clergy, business and civic leaders, environmental activists, state and national organizations, parents, and consumers.

In 1991, the health department was a runner-up for the National Association of County Health Officials' (NACHO; now the National Association of County and City Health Officials or NACCHO) J. Howard Beard Award for community health coalition-building. Most of the Gateway Health Coalition's efforts have been spent in three nontraditional public health–related problem areas: child sexual abuse (now broadened to all child abuse and neglect); the environment (the Gateway Region Environment-Education Network, or GRE-EN, which in 1990 received the first NACHO Environmental Award); and injury control. The health department continues to receive federal Victims of Crime Act funds through the Kentucky Justice Cabinet and a variety of federal Environmental Protection Agency funds from the Cabinet for Natural Resources and Environmental Protection for the GRE-EN programs.

BUILDING AN INITIAL CONSENSUS

The federal Rural Health Outreach Program had funded rural emergency medical service (EMS) systems throughout the nation, but the Gateway EMS systems had been greatly strengthened in four of the five counties (including paramedic training) primarily through the Health Coalition Injury Control Committees. After consultation with the EMS Coordinator and others in the area, I felt that expansion of health and human services in the schools would be the most appropriate action to pursue. At this time, adolescent health units existed in all five county school systems, covering all middle and high schools except one high school in Rowan County. These units served between 77 and 98 percent of the students enrolled in each school. The first step was to convene selected nursing and social work staff and their supervisors from the existing health units, staff who had worked on the Gateway Health Coalition projects, and a representative from the St. Claire Medical Center, the area's largest hospital and primary care clinic complex.

The health department nursing staff vigorously pointed out the major problems they were seeing in the school adolescent units: these included incomplete immunizations, teen pregnancies, low self-esteem, substance abuse (particularly alcohol), violence, truancy, disciplinary referrals, and high drop-out rates. The staff also felt they were badly understaffed to cope with the extent of the problems they faced, and found it difficult to do the prevention screening, which was their primary mandate. They wanted the Rural Health Outreach grant to provide for the development of a unit in Rowan County High School, to increase the nurse staff, and to add social workers to the high school units. (In general, the treatment staff in the middle schools consisted of one nurse per unit and one social worker.)

After further study of the grantor's RFP, I decided that expansion of the existing services would not be acceptable to the grantor. Health department staff, representatives from the hospital and the community mental health system (Pathways), and the director of the Morehead Treatment Center, a center for delinquent girls, were pulled together. A major discussion ensued about the locations and the specifics of the program. The hospital representative pointed out that demographic and health data in Menifee and Morgan counties would make the grant proposal competitive, and he further emphasized that the designation of Menifee County as a health manpower shortage area would meet the RFP requirement that the project be in a rural area with a lack of basic health care services. He also had his own objectives (see below). The director of the Morehead Treatment Center and I felt that a program should be designed that would prevent the problems seen in the adolescent units, when it is often too late for effective treatment.

The group consensus was that the primary objectives should be to do the following:

1. develop a program in the two neediest counties in the region;
2. develop a program in elementary schools (federal funding for maternal and child health care through the state was only available for the adolescent population);
3. identify the elementary schools (it was clear that the maximum funds available would not fund programs in seven elementary schools, five of which were in Morgan and two in Menifee);
4. develop a program not only for the elementary students but also for pre-school children and family members (including pregnant mothers); and
5. pull all the stakeholders together; and develop a consensus on the program details from all players.

STAKEHOLDER ANALYSIS

Another meeting was attended by nursing, social work, and health coalition staff, and representatives from St. Claire Medical Center, Pathways, and from both the Menifee and Morgan County school systems. At this point each group had its own objectives. At the health department level, I felt that the school health units, with their ability to provide health care access to students, would strengthen health department relationships with area providers and be instrumental in bringing health, mental health, human, and educational services together in one site. These integrated services could then provide a continuing role in the rapidly changing health care scene. The health department's provider staff agreed that the proposed plan for a program in elementary schools was worthwhile, but their priority—increasing staff for existing programs—remained. The nursing administrative staff felt that new programs would overburden them and they wanted assistance. Further, the health department's director of administration was somewhat reluctant to take on a large project, which would certainly require much additional effort, for not only would the project require an increase in staff, which would bring about other problems, but it would also necessitate expanded administrative logistics related to developing clinic space, actually setting up the clinics, and maintaining supplies, all at remote sites.

Another primary stakeholder, the St. Claire Medical Center in Rowan County, has for many years been involved in outreach services, receiving the "Outstanding Rural Practice Award for 1993" from the National Rural Health Association. Medical center staff have been heavily involved in the Gateway Health Coalition since its inception and have worked with the health department in a number of specific projects over the years. They brought to this new project an assurance that primary health care and medical specialty care would be available for children and families who might otherwise postpone medical intervention. The medical center representative, however, had an additional set of objectives:

- to continue expanding the center's influence in the community;
- to increase the utilization of the staff in the Menifee primary care clinic (thereby increasing reimbursement to the Medical Center); and
- to increase the center's influence in Morgan County, where most practicing primary care physicians were getting close to retirement and the small county hospital had a need for specialty services such as obstetrics and orthopaedic and vascular surgery.

Pathways, the community mental health center, covers 10 counties in northeast Kentucky, three of which have large industrial bases along the West Virginia border. The Pathways representative had different objectives. When first approached, the director of Pathways became interested in a cooperative agreement. He, too, wanted to increase reimbursement and revenue, but at the time Pathways was just beginning to extend services beyond office walls. The agency had already recognized that schools were in need and were initiating services at school sites in the Gateway area. This project gave Pathways a good opportunity to expand in this direction and gain further acceptance in the community (trust from the Gateway community, particularly the schools, had previously been nonexistent). A major objective was to make sure that all services were reimbursed. Historically, mental health workers had never shared records with other agencies, and one of their objectives was to maintain this confidentiality.

Representatives from the offices of school superintendents for Morgan and Menifee counties attended the organizational meetings as did the Family Resource/Youth Services Center (FRYSC) director in Menifee. Developed through the Kentucky Education Reform Act of 1990, FRYSCs were on-site referral centers primarily for human service needs for children and families. Menifee had some experience with a school-based adolescent health unit by then, and so the county was enthusiastic about extending such services to an outlying elementary school as well as increasing services in the elementary school on the main campus. Perhaps because of the FRYSC in Menifee, the Menifee representative was cognizant of the numbers of dysfunctional families in the county and other problems reflected in area health data, and so he tended to influence the Morgan representative positively. Both schools, however, had severe space limitations and cited solving this problem as a major objective. Both recognized that children who are not healthy or whose family situations are disruptive will not perform well in school, and both were interested in measuring a number of school outcomes in addition to realizing the planned health outcomes.

STRATEGIES

The demographics and needs assessments for both Menifee and Morgan counties as well as the RFP requirements, dictated that these two counties be selected for the project. All stakeholders took part in discussions regarding the choice of schools for the new health units and the specific services to be delivered in those units, though it was clear that both schools in Menifee County should have units. One of these is on the Morgan County line, so consideration was given to developing part-time units in the two small Morgan schools near Menifee. Health department staff concluded that creating the part-time units would be difficult logistically, particularly with a new program. So all agreed that the third school should be in the Morgan County seat, which contained the largest elementary school (418 students). (After implementation of the program and at the request of the school system, one of the two nurses assigned to this unit was transferred to two of the larger outlying elementary schools.)

No one could argue against the desirability of a program in the elementary grades to provide preventive treatment in high-risk situations, in the hope that the severe problems seen in adolescents in the middle and high schools would be ameliorated. Health department staff agreed that this goal was worthwhile, but still resented the fact that they were not going to get help in the existing programs, which was their major objective. As also mentioned, one of the objectives of the nursing administrative staff was to get administrative assistance with the addition of more school health units. Unfortunately, there were insufficient funds available. The school program's nursing supervisor, in particular, has done an extraordinarily capable job; however, she justifiably feels stretched to the limit. Nursing and administrative staff have always been extremely dedicated, so despite their initial resistance, they have fully supported the program.

Another dimension was added to the treatment program when it was decided that all families would be screened for potential high-risk situations by the social worker (provider staff at each site was to include a social worker with a master's degree along with the nurse). The only conflict came up during the implementation phase of the grant, when we discovered that sufficient numbers of qualified social workers did not exist in the area. Health department administrative staff urged the abandonment of the family screening component of the program, which I still strongly supported. The compromise was to hire social workers with bachelor's degrees who could be trained to screen families, but who would have to refer all counseling to the mental health staff. This has worked well.

As mentioned, the medical center representative and I worked together on numerous joint programs over the previous 10 years and we dovetailed easily with the objectives of this project. It was not practical to provide referral services in the school sites since one could never be sure what would be needed or when. To ensure they get needed services, clients are now going to provider sites, and health unit staff now track clients.

The only conflict arose after implementation, when the health department nursing staff heard complaints from clients about the bills they were receiving from the medical center. This presented a situation over which I had no control and I could only suggest that nurses reassure the clients that if they had no money, they would not ultimately be required to pay. Referrals to the private sector in Morgan County were handled in the same way and caused no problem. There have been no complaints from the private sector physicians in either county with regard to competition; in fact, they have received numerous referrals to treat children in need of care, some with serious illnesses.

It was obvious from the beginning that the mental health center would require ultimate reimbursement for all services. It was agreed that the 50 percent services they donated to the project would be those reimbursed by Medicaid and other sources of insurance or payment. The remaining 50 percent was to be paid through the grant. In fact, the State Department for Health Services did not allow the health department to develop a contract with the mental health center during the first year of operation (though the contract was signed for the second year), on the grounds that these services were the mental health center's responsibility. The services were provided as needed during the first year and clearly some were donated to the project. These services were provided at the school sites, an approach that has worked remarkably well. Mental health staff still maintain their own records, which are not open to health department staff. A joint confidentiality release of information form has been developed for signature by the client or parent/guardian; it allows for the exchange of appropriate clinical information between all school-based providers.

A final issue that required resolution was space; neither county school system had an adequate site for the new health units. At the time of the grant request, double-width trailers were included in the budget, one for each of the schools in the respective county seats. The outlying Menifee school had a dental unit that had been used for a number of years by the University of Kentucky College of Dentistry so that their students could treat genuine dental pathology (the College of Dentistry is now a consortium member).

The dental unit, which was under the broad administrative umbrella of the health department, was staffed only one day a week. It was determined that this space could also double for the health unit. The first problem arose when it was discovered that the $8,000 that had been budgeted per secondhand trailer would not begin to cover the purchase cost, while at the same time the Menifee School System decided it did not have appropriate land space for a trailer at their main elementary school site. Menifee wanted to renovate space within the school, but renovation costs were not allowed by the funding agent. The health department's Director of Administrative Services reworked the budget to provide assistance for renovation; implementation of full services was thus delayed longer than expected. Toyota Motor Manufacturing donated a modular building (a simple shell with no divisions into rooms) to the Morgan school; again, the health department budget was stretched to cover extremely high renovation costs. Fortunately, significant funds were available from the delay in hiring staff, and permission to use these was granted by the funding agency. This unit was finally ready in December 1995, 16 months after the grant award. Since January 1995, services had been delivered in a cramped space next to the school's stage. Both school systems willingly donated phones, office supplies, copying capability, etc., to the project.

With the advent of "Teen Initiative Projects" and health education programs (including "family living" education) initiated by health department staff, in 1986 the health department had begun to work with parents, teachers, school councils, and school system superintendents in all five county school systems. These persons reviewed in detail all health education curricula and helped to develop the consent forms that would be signed by all parents or guardians; they were also fully informed on all aspects of the school programs as they were developed, including the adolescent health units. Discussions included policies and procedures, protocols, and more complicated consent forms. These same processes were used in the development of this elementary school project, and formal approvals were obtained from the appropriate school councils (made up of teachers and school principals as well as parents) for the program as well as for the multiagency (health department and mental health) consent forms. By the time the elementary school project came along, these community members were aware of the benefits of the adolescent health units and no conflicts could be identified.

DISCUSSION

This project, now known as the Rural Outreach Program for Elementary Students (ROPES), was awarded a three-year grant by the federal Rural Health Outreach Grant Program in September 1994. The program has been so successful that the four-county school districts who do not have services at all schools—only Menifee is covered—have requested coverage. This would mean the addition of services to 12 more elementary schools and to the high school in Rowan County, bringing the total to 26 units.

Within a few months after the elementary health units had opened, staff began to recognize the extent to which children's health care is neglected in Appalachia. It was discovered that these children have not been receiving adequate medical care, much less preventive health care. For example, despite a state law requiring complete immunization on entry into school, 25 children needed immunizations when the first unit opened. At another school, 32 children were found to have abnormal vision; of these, five received glasses. There were also 13 children whose hearing screenings were abnormal and two from this group received hearing aids.

Some case studies indicate the program's effectiveness. A seven-year-old girl with severe asthma was experiencing frequent asthma attacks, which often kept her from school. Her parents worked, did not have health insurance, and were not eligible for Medicaid. They were sometimes unable to purchase the prescription asthma medications and inhalers the child needed. The child received a well-child exam at the school health unit and was referred to the Regional Pediatrics Program, which is staffed by a pediatrician from a large private medical clinic in the health department center in Rowan County. The child's medication schedule was changed and newer medications were given, with the program paying for the child's medications. The child has experienced a 70 percent decrease in the incidence of asthma attacks and an improvement in overall health. She now has good attendance at school and improved academic performance. An eight-year-old boy with attention deficit disorder who was in a learning disability class was seen by this same health unit. The child had frequent upper respiratory, sinus, and ear infections. The child was referred to the Commission for Children with Special Health Care Needs, housed in health department facilities in Rowan County, and now has ear tubes. At present, he is making great academic progress and is no longer in the learning disability class. Previously, he was quiet and withdrawn, but since being given ear tubes, he is more outgoing.

At another school, a six-year-old student was referred to the health unit nurse by a school bus driver when the student became unable to lift his leg to get on the bus (the mother thought the child had growing pains). The nurse referred the child to his family physician, who referred him to an orthopaedic specialist. The diagnosis of Perthes' disease was made, and the child was fitted for a brace. The health unit nurse not only made the appropriate referral but also contacted funding agencies for payment for these services. In another example, a five-year-old student came to school, became ill and started vomiting. He was diagnosed with meningococcal meningitis, a highly infectious illness, and was hospitalized. The school health unit nurse assisted the health department nurse in identifying contacts and dispensing prophylactic medication. Home visits were made and approximately 50 persons received such medication. There were no new cases identified. These are just a few of the cases exemplifying the health problems and their treatment in the Gateway area. Despite the availability of medical care services in the area, they are not necessarily readily accessible.

Though several problems with collaborative efforts have been described in the development of ROPES, these were not insurmountable, and all stakeholders have been pleased with the results. I believe that the relative ease with which this new outreach was accomplished is directly due to the approximately 10-year history of collaborative efforts in the area, through both the Gateway Health Coalition and the various programs within the schools. Each stakeholder had concerns regarding the internal functions of his or her agency, but "turf" and "trust" were never issues because of the long history of collaboration between provider agencies among school systems. Each stakeholder felt free to communicate ideas and concerns, thereby helping to maintain the collaborative atmosphere.

Since the award of the grant, there have been regular stakeholder meetings to monitor progress and suggest modifications, and the general atmosphere of cooperation remains unchanged. This process is nurtured by health department feedback to the stakeholders of problems, successes achieved, special anecdotes, etc. Though the project is administered by the health department, the agency has continued to act primarily as the communicator, coordinator, and convener throughout, in accordance with the roles developed through 10 years of coalition building in Gateway. In this particular project, I served as facilitator in the development of the project and continue to do so in the follow-up meetings, though I officially retired in August 1994.

Generally in this process, which must be continually open at all levels, effective communication is perhaps the most difficult. As the health department staff member primarily responsible for the development of the school programs has recently said, "Everything has to be on the top of the table at all times, for anything under the table destroys trust. Trust is very fragile." For me, it has also meant stepping out of the physician's authoritarian role and addressing collaborative efforts and supporting joint decisions, both among staff and members of the community. On occasion too, particularly in my dealing with persons from remote Appalachia, I have learned that gender and accent sometimes put one at an initial disadvantage in leading the discussions, so others were sometimes delegated to communicate with individuals from a markedly different culture.

Acting as an agent for change is not without risk, but the results can be rewarding. In the ultraconservative atmosphere of Appalachia, physicians are expected to provide clinical services. Through the years, several pressing community health problems have been addressed, additional resources have been brought into the area, and the health department has received national accolades. Yet in reality my sole monetary value to the board of health has been as a clinician, rather than as an administrator. Family planning in the five Gateway counties, and tuberculosis screening and treatment in an additional 10 counties, has had to take priority. Personal rewards, however, have been far greater in the areas of coalition building and in the development of integrated delivery of services. My management style as a physician commissioner of health has been to delegate the business administration to the health department administrator and to pull together the management team members, which include administrator, clinical/environmental service directors, and Gateway Health Coalition staff, for brainstorming sessions and joint team decisions on new directions to take in the pursuit of better meeting community needs.

The outcomes realized from this particular project have made all the stakeholders feel good about the program. In fact, these same stakeholders, plus representatives of another hospital, other public services (social services and welfare/entitlement services), the other three school systems, Morehead State University, the Gateway area development district, and representatives from the court system, local industry and community leaders, county government, political leaders, and consumers will form the governing board of a new collaborative effort, through which it is hoped that all health and human services as well as educational and support services can be integrated and delivered collaboratively in the Gateway area.

The project, known as the Gateway Region Interagency Delivery System was one of four to win a technical assistance award from the Kentucky Commission on Families and Children; it may take several years to implement fully. Currently, I serve as the acting chairman of this group and will continue to do so until it is further along in its development. Since I am no longer employed by an agency, I am perceived as a neutral individual without turf concerns. Because of this perception, I have the ability to negotiate more freely, particularly with state officials. At the same time, there exists the challenge of ensuring a smooth transition to a permanently functioning organization under new, dynamic, and appropriate leadership. This will not be carried out by any single individual but rather through the collaborative efforts of a committed team.

CHAPTER 11

Repositioning a State Health Agency in an Era of Change through Developing the Internal Customer: A Case Study in Leadership

Kaye W. Bender

> To keep our faces toward change and behave like free spirits in the presence of fate is strength undefeatable.
>
> —*Helen Keller*

I am a 19-year veteran of the public health system in Mississippi. Like many others who have chosen public health as their specialty, I have grown up in the system, enthusiastically participating in activities at many levels within the public health organization of the Mississippi State Department of Health. I have had many wonderful opportunities to grow and learn, and I have been faced with equally as many challenges and struggles. Like many other Mississippi public health workers, this is my home state, and my interests center around doing what I can to make it a healthier place to live and work.

Mississippi was one of the states selected for site visitation when the Institute of Medicine decided to conduct a study on the future of public health. Many of the conclusions and recommendations that resulted from that study apply to our state, and it remains a pleasant experience to thumb through the book and see the reality of public health in Mississippi reflected so well.[1] One aspect, however, had been foreign to us. The report describes all too well the short tenure of most of the state health commissioners around the country. It also addresses the fragmented nature

With consultation from NancyKay Sullivan Wessman, Director, Health Communications, Mississippi State Department of Health and Linda H. Potts, School of Public Health, University of Alabama at Birmingham.

of public health planning and policy development at a time when leadership does not have the opportunity to complete the public health system's mission in making sure that change was accomplished. The problem was finding short-term leadership. Our agency could not see that as a difficulty, since continuity is a great strength of the Mississippi public health system. We are almost 120 years old and during this period we have had only six state health officers. Stability has been a way of life. We have been fortunate to see our public health system remain intact long enough to experience the benefits of many policy decisions and the changes in systems designs we have made.

This case study is being written to describe what happens when that stability is threatened, whether in a real or perceived sense, and how management staff have an opportunity to call on their leadership skills to address some of the issues and concerns associated with change in an organization. In essence, the question facing us was, "At a time when the entire health care system is being threatened with the chaos of change, how can a state with a long history of stability and continuity maintain the best of what it has, while looking ahead to adopt the best of what is to be?"

HISTORICAL CONTEXT

Mississippi, one of the Deep South states along the Gulf of Mexico, is primarily a rural state. It has 82 counties occupying almost 48,000 square miles. The population of the state is approximately 2.5 million persons, representing a population density of 54.2 persons per square mile. Only seven of the 82 counties are included as Standard Metropolitan Statistical Areas, and these seven counties are located in three geographical areas. There are 290 incorporated cities, villages, and towns. The state has experienced a 2.6 percent population gain in the past decade.

The demography of the state contributes significantly to its history. The population is 63.5 percent Caucasian, 35.6 percent African American, and one percent other races. Mississippi has consistently been at the low end of the diverse socioeconomic and health profile of the United States. It ranks lowest among the states for income level, with a median household income for a family of four totaling less than $20,000. Only 30 of the 82 counties have 50 percent of the residents graduating from high school. With education attainment at that level, it is not surprising that unemployment levels rank among the top three in the nation. Mississippi also ranks next to last among the southeastern states in expenditures for health care. Approximately 467,000 persons in the state are uninsured and depend on the public system, along with those hospitals and other health providers who are willing to provide for their care. The state also has the lowest ranking for physician-to-population ratio.

The Mississippi State Department of Health was formed in 1877. It is an agency that is governed by a 13-member board, appointed by the governor for staggered terms. The state health officer is appointed by and is accountable to the State

Board of Health. The department is a totally centralized organization that is administered by the state health officer. A network of 110 full-time public health clinics, 26 regional home health offices, and 93 Women's, Infants' and Children's Program Distribution Centers covers the entire state. There are 3,000 employees, all agents of the state, who are distributed among the counties and regions and carry out the mission of the agency. Statutorily, the department has the authority to administer services and programs in a broad range of areas, such as maternal-child health, environmental health (individual on-site wastewater, public water supply, milk regulation, food sanitation, radiological health, and boiler pressure vessel safety), family planning, control of communicable diseases (including sexually transmitted diseases), newborn genetic screening, well-child health services, immunizations, tuberculosis control, licensure of 16 different health professions, health facilities licensure and certification, and certificate of need for health planning.

The state has historically provided a significant amount of clinic-based primary and preventive health services (for example, 52% of all prenatal care in the state is provided by the state agency). We have spent a lot of time and energy over the past 20 years focusing on the internal standards of care and in ensuring that services are standardized throughout the state. We have been proud of the fact that one could visit any county health department in the state at any time and basically see the same menu of service delivery and standard of care. Our time and emphasis have been spent in developing protocols, program standards, and quality assurance and fiscal audit capability. Program and fiscal integrity are valued by the staff.

In 1993, we were faced with a new challenge: the hiring of a new state health officer. Unlike the majority of the states described in the Institute of Medicine study, Mississippi had enjoyed the stability of having one health officer at the helm for over 20 years. That alone presented a significant challenge to the staff, for to face that change in the wake of health care reform made for an unusually difficult situation. The executive management team of the agency originally felt the weight of the responsibility to attempt to make the internal change, brought about by the hiring of the state health officer, as well as the external change resulting from reform in the health care system, as transparent to the staff throughout the agency as possible. However, that goal was neither logical nor practical. It was, however, the impetus for the beginning of one of the most educational experiences with which we have been involved. Embracing the need to change with the times, we felt a sense of responsibility in regard to the new state health officer and the 3,000 coworkers that called us into action. We needed a plan, a new vision for the future.

INITIAL PHASE

Initially, the agency contracted with the University of Alabama School of Public Health and a local marketing firm to develop a communication/information plan that would facilitate the repositioning of the agency in the face of changes expected to occur under health care reform. During the designing of the project, however, the national emphasis on health care reform became dormant even as the changes in the health care delivery system were continuing to evolve incrementally. These changes, though slower to occur than in many other states, included the mandate for Medicaid managed care, an unusual growth in the number and distribution of rural health clinics throughout the state (from seven to 142 in a two-year period), and the potential for establishing a health planning authority.

Although we knew by this time that the new chief would be chosen from among the staff itself, many of the employees were having difficulty separating the national and state pictures. There was also unrest with the external changes brought upon the agency in response to the new administration policies and procedures. The contractor was asked to shift the focus of the study slightly to address the issues as they arose. We determined at this point to recognize that the internal customers had to be developed as quickly as possible for the agency to remain healthy in the wake of these changes. We felt, and the contractors concurred, that creating an internal constituency should precede focusing on any external support that was going to be needed in the future.

PHASE II

The project team met with members of the state health officer's staff early in the process. At that time, the scope of the project was redefined to include employees within the department. External constituencies, such as health policy decision makers, would not be included until a later date. Information was provided to the team, which outlined past strategies and activities related to communications and information management. Other documents such as organizational charts were made available as well. A series of interviews with agency personnel, including a sample of field office administrators, were conducted. In total, 25 individuals were involved in this phase of the project.

The interviews were used to create an internal scan of the agency. Relevant factors for inclusion in the final plan were identified. These factors included such items as the staff's perceptions of the agency's organizational issues, its leadership position within the state as a whole, the existence of strategic alliances at a state and federal level, public relations capabilities, the position of leadership with respect to legislative and policy-making bodies, and past communication strategies that had been successful in managing change. Of particular importance within this part of the process was the state health officer's "vision" for the future of the agency. An external scan provided information in factors that might affect the success of the plan. These factors included items such as perceptions related to the agency's mission as well as political, economic, social, and technological factors that might impact on national and statewide data related to plan development and successful implementation.

RESULTS

Raw data from these interviews yielded some interesting, useful results. The internal assessment covered concerns such as reductions in revenue streams and the resulting uncertainty and lack of understanding of the new state health officer's mission and vision for the agency. There was also a very real sense of urgency regarding the provision of some of the direct care services, both for potential premature loss of care for patients and for potential individual job loss. Additionally, there was a fair amount of concern expressed that all this change was not needed and that the management staff could do something about it if we chose to do so.

The external survey reminded us of a number of problems: the five-year personnel reduction plan mandated by the state legislature; the lack of understanding by the public as well as by some of our staff about what the agency does; the need to make a firm decision about our role in the provision of direct care services under the Medicaid managed care contracts; and the need to work more closely with our local community partners.

In many ways, these surveys told us what we thought we knew, namely, that we had a big job ahead in planning for the future. They also told us some things that we didn't know. We were unaware, for example, of the level of uncertainty that our staff throughout the state felt in regard to the upcoming change. After consolidating the findings of the interviews, we conducted strategic reviews to analyze the findings for a fit with the agency's mission, goals, and plans for management of change. A small focus group of selected agency personnel representing both central office and field staff helped the project team identify strengths and weaknesses related to the agency's communications and information systems; participants identified and set priorities for components of the proposed communications plan.

The team identified several objectives for the public health administration's focus, such as a clear emphasis on the core functions of public health. We also identified problems and acknowledged the difficulty of building a strong tax base for prevention based on the awareness that data related to prevention are soft compared to data on clinic patients served. We recognized that the employees as well as the public are generally uninformed about public health technologies. The same group suggested ways the agency could maximize opportunities and overcome weaknesses that could be threats or barriers to implementation. Strategies gathered from this process form the basis of the proposed plan.

Strengths identified through the surveys included the acknowledgment that agency leadership enjoys strong support, that this period of change was in all probability a unique window of opportunity, and that public health staff throughout the state are viewed as respected professionals with high credibility. We were also reminded that since we are a statewide organization, our public health work force could be viewed as our greatest asset.

Weaknesses were pointed out. They included the acknowledgment that a corporate culture is not conducive to change, that our work force is limited in policy analysis and formulation skills, and that many personnel lack professional training in public health and prevention and may not understand core functions of public health.

The state health officer and his staff studied the information gathered during the interviews and focus groups; we reviewed strategies, rationales, proposed models, and recommendations for development of a communications plan to facilitate the repositioning of the agency. From this review, four major recommendations were made.

1. Leadership objectives and the direction of the agency should be communicated to all personnel. This would be achieved through statewide staff meeting via a satellite-based communications system, through personal appearances, and through the strategic planning process.
2. Employees should be educated about the upcoming reform. Strategies to achieve this goal include a seminar series for statewide and district-based leaders, more participation in regional and national public health meetings, distance learning, and an employee newsletter to focus on agency direction, core public health functions, and other issues relevant to the work force.
3. Plans for managing change should be established. Such plans would incorporate a comprehensive strategic planning process, interdisciplinary planning and information sharing sessions, and the task forces' development of suggestions for strategic planning consideration, including employee communications, staff development, new mission/values, partnerships, new money, and information systems.
4. Legislators and other decision makers should be educated about upcoming changes. To this end, formal alliances should be made with education, economic development, and other health care organizations. Periodic communications with legislators and other public officials, annual public health legislative conferences, and alliances and contracts with businesses can all be useful in making reform known.

With all of this information now available to us, it was clear that the need for developing an internal constituency was far greater than the need to develop a communications plan. Knowing the organization's history at various levels, and cognizant of the external exposure as well, I felt keenly that our task was significant. We had to figure out how to create an internal constituency in order to determine both what we needed to keep in the face of this change and what we needed to change in order to excel in the new health care environment.

The state health officer, Dr. F.E. Thompson, held the first-ever statewide staff meeting via teleconference and shared his view of the future, extending a challenge to the staff throughout the state to distinguish between health care and public health. He also prepared the staff for the changing nature of the business and encouraged them to consider that standardization of health care services statewide would no longer be the focus; instead, meeting the public health needs of each local community would be. For the first time in several years, county health departments throughout the state would be encouraged to continue providing certain services (until a solid provider of care could be identified) or to focus specifically on providing core public health services (assuming there were ample providers for the personal health care services to be found).

The stage was set; the challenge was clear. As staff members in leadership positions, and as believers in promulgating the public health system in Mississippi, we picked up the gauntlet and proceeded to set into motion a process whereby these changes could be discussed, planned, and ultimately evaluated.

The unit directors from the state health officer's staff, under my coordination as chief of the state health officer's staff, served as facilitators for each of the work groups recommended by the contractors. Management staff at the district level solicited membership from the state as a whole. The process of selecting and organizing the work groups took several weeks. A great deal of attention was given to constructing interdisciplinary work groups that reflected the public health work force in Mississippi.

Once the groups were chosen, all groups met for the first time on the same day. The state health officer opened by stating the need for reform and used a vision map developed by the agency artist to start the discussions. I followed his opening comments with a description of the process of change, emphasizing that the work groups each had a mission to accomplish. I indicated that we needed to develop recommendations for specific areas by the fall of 1995, when the strategic planning retreat would take place.

Each group was assured that their recommendations would reach the strategic planning process and that they would receive feedback about the inclusion of those recommendations in the overall plan. I had the privilege of being present at the meetings of all the groups, and I observed a complex array of group dynamics. Two reactions were readily observable: anxiety about being on an advisory committee and doubt that any of the recommendations would ever be used. As the groups continued to meet, however, the discussions soon centered on how the changes might affect the work environment. It also became clear to all of the facilitators that there would be some operational issues that required discussion before we could begin fulfillment of the vision. We were painfully reminded that creating opportunities for dialogue meant that our discussions were basically speculative in nature and that any efforts to move too quickly would not ultimately succeed. We were continuing to learn, not only about the subject at hand, but also about our organizational culture and its dynamics. It was truly a historically important period for the agency, but it will probably be years before the benefits are realized.

Three months later, the management staff held a one-day strategic planning session to hear recommendations from each work group. The session was facilitated by a management consultant from another school of public health. Both strategic and operational issues were identified for inclusion in the agency's strategic plan. The dynamics in that session were very similar to those we had experienced in the small work groups. We were now aware from our interviews that we had reached an internally consistent outlook. We were hearing loud, consistent messages from the original focus groups and from management staff as well. It was time to move forward in the change process and produce some observable results.

OUTCOMES

The effective reorganization of the central office structure decentralizes programs and power, reemphasizes training for the public health work force, and shifts priorities and people to meet emerging needs. Dr. Thompson promised to train and re-train public health workers to provide old-fashioned public health, that is, to do different things in different ways with different techniques. The new design, the first significant one for the agency in 12 years, was created by a committee of management team members which I chaired. It reflects the core functions of public health as well as a flatter organizational chart.

Matching the beginning of that new organizational structure, we introduced the first issue of our new Communicating Opportunities/Reaching Employees (CORE) employee newsletter, which communicates to working people the public health agency's core functions. First published in 1995, the newsletter introduces the work force to public health concepts developed by other leaders and organizations nationwide. We imitate the tactics of the American Public Health Association, the Association of State and Territorial Health Officials and its affiliates, and U.S. Public Health Service leaders—that is, we collect and redistribute written materials and graphics that can equip us in Mississippi to communicate better about what public health is and how we do it in Mississippi. We also look to communications advisors throughout the agency to help select, develop, and publish articles of interest to CORE readers. Since the idea was conceived, we have distributed eight issues. Dr. Thompson says we are "going back to doing what public health does best and nobody else can do: assessment, policy development, and assurance to influence people's health and the quality of our lives" (staff conference, 1 August 1993).

District management staff and state level office directors are involved as a policy advisory team for the agency director. This team is involved in making all policy and creating some of the procedures that affect the agency as a whole. A number of their activities and responsibilities are strategic, and others are operational in nature. However, Dr. Thompson has made the decision that no policy affecting the field operations will be approved without the team's input and advice.

Several work groups have remained intact as advisory committees to their respective areas of expertise. This process has enabled state-level staff working on implementation of the various projects or activities to receive feedback as to the relevance of their work. It also ensures ongoing dialogue between the state level staff and the field staff.

A committee has been established to evaluate the agency's operational planning process. The emphasis has changed from producing documents to establishing an interactive process for leading and managing public health activities in the wake of change. The vision of the group is still in the formative stage, but its underlying philosophy is to foster communication, collaboration, and team-based evaluation of the agency's programs and activities.

LESSONS LEARNED

Most of the activities identified in the process thus far have been productive experiences for the staff who have actively participated in all of the phases of change. However, the unit directors who served as agency leaders in the process have experienced some frustrations along the way. A review of these problems would reasonably serve to guide others about to embark on a similar process (or any other process involving major change) as areas to consider in their initial planning phase.

- As stated previously, the focus of the contract changed early in the process from the development of a communications plan for public health undergoing reform to formulating an overall strategic plan and providing a communications plan under new agency management. We were well into the process before we realized that we had not adequately communicated that shift in focus to the members of the management team. We lost both credibility and time in the process as we had to backtrack to cover the change in focus. We had to learn to value the process as much or more than the product.
- It is hard to differentiate change in management style occurring at the same time that significant external changes are taking place. As leaders, we needed to spend some time preparing our staff for active participation in long-range planning. Doing so would have increased their effectiveness and decreased their frustration. We also think that the level of trust among the group would be increased.
- It is essential to maintain communication throughout the realization of the vision, and so commitment and appreciation and need for staff involvement

are very necessary. We found that we spent a lot of time affirming the significance of the planning process.

- Working with two schools of public health was a productive opportunity for a state with little experience in that regard. However, we have recognized the divergence of backgrounds in formulating assumptions. Again, spending some additional planning and reviewing time on the front end of the process would have made time we did spend together more profitable.
- Many of the staff and also the facilitator of the strategic planning session were surprised that, while strengths, weaknesses, opportunities, and threats were identified in the preliminary sessions held by the work groups and during the session, some topics were not mentioned. Notably, managed care, competition, the agency's position on the provision of direct services, the agency's position on certificate of need, quality management, outcomes, influence in other community sectors, and respect for employees and citizens as resources were not trends noted in the strategic planning session.

At the time of this writing, Mississippi is still developing formal strategic and operational plans. However, the beginning phases of participatory decision making have created an environment in which issues can be addressed in a straightforward manner. I am gradually becoming aware that the final plan is not the object of this exercise at all; the creation of an internal constituency occurs as a learning environment grows and is nurtured. There is truly a great deal of energy to be harnessed if we work to blend reality with vision. This can be achieved by maintaining frank, open communication with regard to policy development and by strongly retaining a sense of the past even as we develop a framework for the future. The process may not be over, but I feel that we have grown a lot simply because it was begun. We are seeing new opportunities for leadership emerge among various members of our staff, and we expect to see more as the dialogue continues. The ultimate beneficiaries will be the public, because our services, however they are to be defined, will be the result of a shared vision of the future for public health in Mississippi.

REFERENCE

1. Institute of Medicine. *The Future of Public Health.* Washington, DC: National Academy Press, 1988.

PART V

The Future

CHAPTER 12

Public Health Practice Guidelines: A Case Study

Lloyd F. Novick

In the autumn of 1993, the Council on Linkages met in San Francisco. This half-day meeting was timed to coincide with a concurrent meeting of the American Public Health Association (APHA). Several years earlier the Council had been formed to bridge the gap between public health practice and academic research. On the agenda was consideration of the merits of the Council's involvement in developing guidelines for public health practice. Guidelines had been determined at several previous Council meetings. Enthusiasm for this initiative was evident, but several observers suspected that contentiousness and control issues were also associated with this proposal. As events unfolded over the next several months, these observations proved correct.

The Council on Linkages consists of representatives from the major organizations representing public health practice and academia. Representatives include those from the Association of State and Territorial Health Officials (ASTHO), the National Association of County Health Officials (NACHO), and the APHA. From the academic sector, members include the American College of Preventive Medicine (ACPM), the American Teachers of Preventive Medicine (ATPM), and the Association of Schools of Public Health (ASPH). The Centers for Disease Control and Prevention (CDC) and Human Resources Service Administration (HRSA) complete the membership.

Guidelines for public health practice were advanced as a concept analogous to guidelines for clinical prevention. Could improved guidance be provided for public health practice by the development of guidelines? Was there a scientific basis for the guidelines similar to that employed by clinical preventive guidelines?

As chair of the council and as a public health practitioner, I recognized the appeal of developing public health guidelines. The process of development would be invaluable and exciting because it required the convening of multidisciplinary groups to work out community health approaches. The issue of guidelines cut to

135

the heart of the question of what formed the basis for public health practice. Can the public health approach be codified? Is it science based? Would guidelines add to the effectiveness of public health activities?

The promise of public health practice guidelines rests in their ability to enhance the translation of scientific advances into community practice. Immunization has been demonstrated to be efficacious, but its actual application is deficient, with low immunization rates for two-year-olds resulting in increased rates of vaccine-preventable disease.

Congenital syphilis can be prevented by testing the mother in prenatal care and by administering penicillin. But the application of this intervention is unsatisfactory in areas such as New York City, where more than 1,000 cases of congenital syphilis occur each year. Again, this high rate can be attributed to the lack of an effective approach, complicated by the major social and substance abuse problems of a vulnerable population.

Council discussion in San Francisco centered on the role of practice guidelines as a future focus of activity. The debate was spirited, but no one would have predicted the extent to which this issue was to remain controversial, or that it would remain a major item on the Council's agenda for the next several years.

Advocates of public health practice guidelines often used clinical guidelines as a comparison. Although this analogy is imperfect, prior experience with clinical preventive guidelines did influence the debate on guidelines for public health practice. In 1989, the *Guide to Clinical Preventive Services* was published under the supervision of the United States Preventive Services Task Force. Dr. Michael McGinnis, Deputy Assistant Secretary of the Department of Health and Human Services, played a prominent role in organizing this effort and was also prominent five years later in shaping public health practice guidelines. Dr. William Wiese of the University of New Mexico was on the Preventive Task Force, and later became the ATPM representative on the Council on Linkages. The perspectives of both these individuals were important to the ongoing discussion of how to develop practice guidelines.

An earlier guide to clinical preventive services was based on scientific evidence that had been rigorously reviewed. It included 169 interventions to prevent 60 different illnesses and conditions. The guide was the culmination of more than four years of literature review, debate, and synthesis of critical comments from expert reviewers. The best judgment of task force members formed the basis for clinical recommendations for preventive services.

A 1976 effort similarly emphasized a scientific basis for evaluating clinical preventive services. The Canadian government convened a task force to study the periodic health examination. This expert panel used a highly structured approach to evaluating the effectiveness of clinical preventive services. Explicit criteria were developed to judge the quality of evidence from published clinical research.

Uniform decision-making rules were used to evaluate the strength of preventive recommendations.

THE DEBATE

During the next two years, the Council debated what priority to assign to the development of practice guidelines. Regular participants were Council members and observers, notably staff of the U.S. Public Health Service (PHS). While there was overall agreement that practice guidelines were worthy of exploration and certainly of continued discussion, considerable controversy was generated over such questions as how to proceed or, indeed, whether to proceed at all with their development.

Of primary concern was the extent to which public health practice guidelines could be expected to have a scientific basis and therefore be analogous to the earlier efforts establishing clinical and preventive recommendations. The absence of scientific studies backing public health interventions was seen as an impediment. Guidelines based on expert opinion were not favored.

An additional obstacle was the nature of public health practice and the character of community health issues. Members of the council commented that these issues are often dissimilar from clinical issues. Public health problems are multifactorial in nature, with social, educational, and economic components. A problem such as congenital syphilis does not result only from an infectious agent; it is related to substance abuse, prenatal care, and lack of educational attainment. How could a guideline be constructed for broad-based problems stemming from multiple social ills? There was also the problem of addressing the extent to which a generic guideline would be adequate for widely divergent communities in disparate locations.

Some of the sharpest questioning of the guideline concept came from representatives of the PHS. How were these new guidelines different from the information already disseminated by the CDC? For example, the CDC provides a wealth of guidance on immunization, tuberculosis, and sexually transmitted disease. The number of such guidelines available from the CDC was reported to be about 40 in the beginning. As the debate about the new guidelines' usefulness continued, the CDC identified more than 200 others it had developed.

Questions came up about who would develop and control the public health guidelines. Clearly the Council's interest in the subject was stimulating the interest of federal health agencies in identifying more and more guidelines. It was not clear whether official federal health agencies were to be assigned this responsibility or whether local public health practitioners would also be involved.

Even the format of the guidelines became an item of dispute. The chair of the council and others preferred health problems as the focus suitable for guidelines.

Public health service representatives preferred that the format be similar to the list of essential public health functions. Preparing a guideline for a generic function, such as community mobilization or outreach, as compared to more specific guidance for a disease or health problem, such as prevention of cardiovascular disease, required a different approach.

Discussion continued at Council meetings over the next year. The debate had several planes. Practitioners wanted practice guidelines. Academics were also interested in the potential of this initiative, but they only wanted to proceed if there was a scientific base. Federal participation raised a number of the technical and feasibility issues, yet underlying them was the question of control. Would a nongovernmental group now assume the mission of providing public health guidance? And, alternatively, if the federal health agencies were to assume this development responsibility, would they be saddled with too large a task? What was the priority for this venture, which would clearly be resource intensive?

The Council's chair saw federal involvement as necessary because of the resources it required. Local collaboration, also needed, had to be defined. Discussions continued, but no decision was made on future specific actions. The Council decided on an independent planning effort, because Council members felt that such an effort would catalyze the various players and stimulate federal involvement. The W.K. Kellogg Foundation, already familiar with council discussions, was approached by the chair. In response to his request, the foundation agreed to provide $150,000 for a planning effort. This grant would enable the council to examine the two principle issues that had emerged during the debate: the adequacy of scientific evidence for public health interventions; and the feasibility and desirability of implementing guidelines for public health practice.

THE PUBLIC HEALTH PRACTICE GUIDELINE DEVELOPMENT PROJECT

As the Council chair, I met with Ron Bialek, staff director, to decide on a course of action, one with the best chance of success in stimulating the eventual development of these practice guidelines. Agreement was reached on a number of issues:

1. Our efforts would attempt to provide documentation for the need or absence of need for practice guidelines. The project would not develop final guidelines, as neither the resources nor time period allocated were sufficient to do so.
2. Our method would employ specific queries that focused on particular health problems. These queries would serve as examples or tracers of subjects for potential guidelines.
3. We would examine two issues raised by the previous debate. First, was there an adequate scientific base for the generation of practice guidelines in public

health? Second, how did practitioners and other experts view the creation of this type of guideline in terms of feasibility, implementation, and resultant benefits?

The project was to be directed by myself. We set up a subcontract for staff work with the Health Program Alliance (HPA) at Johns Hopkins University. The Council on Linkages was advisory to the project. In this way, we gained considerable autonomy in the administration of the project, and oversight was provided by the council.

Four public health challenges were chosen for study. They included complete and timely immunization of preschool children, completion of treatment for tuberculosis, prevention of cardiovascular disease, and prevention of lead poisoning in children. I selected these problems for study because they represented likely opportunities for gathering information on factors important to guideline development. They were in many ways a cross-section of major population-based interventions. The health issues encompassed prevention and treatment, community outreach and targeted subgroups, defined diseases and a diversity of risk factors, and medical solutions and environmental reforms.

The strategy of the leaders was to examine the feasibility of evidence-based practice guidelines for this group of issues. If evidence-based practice guidelines were deemed feasible for this cross-section of public health challenges, they would be feasible for many other public health challenges as well.

An expert in each of the four areas was selected to chair a multidisciplinary panel that would examine the evidence and the feasibility for practice guidelines. A resident specializing in preventive medicine or a graduate student in public health was also chosen to assist for the staff work. The panels were completed by invitations to nine to 12 public health experts knowledgeable about population-based interventions. In addition to primary care physicians, panel members included representatives of federal, state, and local health agencies; managed care and other private health organizations; academic institutions; community organizations; and voluntary associations.

Each panel was charged with answering three questions:

1. Is there enough evidence of sufficient quality now available to support the development of public health practice guidelines?
2. Are the practice guidelines desirable and feasible?
3. Should the task of developing practice guidelines be undertaken now?

The co-directors had designed a project that required only minimal resources but would address the key questions for the four conditions we had chosen to focus on. Further, by involving a broad array of national experts, the co-directors were assured of authoritative advice and maximum visibility for the findings.

SEARCH FOR EVIDENCE

Assembling the relevant literature in each area of concern required a major effort. After a preliminary review of the procedures employed in successful programs to develop clinical guidelines, HPA staff developed a pilot method for identifying, screening, and collecting the appropriate literature for the panels' more detailed review.

Literature was first identified through searches of *Medline* and other electronic databases. Inquiries requesting selected references were then made to authorities in each topic area and to selected state health departments.

To sort the mass of accumulating literature, two methods were employed. One was to match data against a standard list of 10 essential public health services. Also, for each area the director and panel chairs developed a set of critical questions, highlighting queries that needed to be answered by the guidelines. Critical questions were not meant to comprehensively define any one guideline. They were a limited tool for the pilot study to assess the adequacy of the available evidence. Each item of literature was then assigned to one or more critical questions, and the questions and associated literature were allocated to panel members for review.

The panels and preventive medicine residents approached the task of literature review with vigor. For cardiovascular disease, the *Medline* search retrieved over 33,000 citations, of which 3,181 were determined to be relevant. Eventually, 220 articles were assigned to this database. Later, when actual guideline development began, this database proved invaluable.

BALTIMORE MEETING

In April 1995 the directors, the four teams, the HPA staff, and invited observers gathered in Baltimore. There the work was divided between panel sessions—each panel sought consensus on the evidence and the feasibility and desirability of guidelines—and plenary sessions, in which the panels shared their conclusions. As the meeting progressed, participants expressed enthusiasm about the prospect of practice guidelines and remarked repeatedly about the advantages of working on public health problems with the perspectives provided by the multidisciplinary panels.

All four expert panels were in agreement that evidence-based guidelines for public health practice are feasible, and each panel recommended that such guidelines be developed for its program area. Each panel independently concluded that a well-directed effort to write and implement such guidelines would be justified by the potential benefits, which were seen as immediate and far reaching at every stage of the public health process. For problems that required action, the guidelines would suggest effective strategies and interventions, recommend priorities for efficient use of resources, and provide benchmarks for broad policy. Evidence-based guidelines would also enhance the legitimacy of public health activities.

The meeting concluded with overwhelming support for further development of the guidelines. The leaders were pleased with the result, knowing the substantive and strategic value of a strong endorsement on the part of public health experts. After this meeting, the leaders followed up with renewed approaches to the U.S. PHS. While this proved helpful, more efforts in tandem with the various public health constituencies that had attended the meeting would have gathered strengthened support for the guideline concept and would have provided a needed boost for future development.

CONTINUED PROGRESS

Shortly after the meeting in Baltimore, the leaders were invited to a meeting of public health service agency chiefs, chaired by Phil Lee, Assistant Secretary for Health and Human Services. After the presentation of the findings of the Public Health Development Project, a spirited discussion ensued. Both Lee and David Satcher, Director of the CDC, expressed enthusiasm for development of public health practice guidelines. The group discussed its commitment to assist in the implementation of the guidelines. Other agency heads were also interested, requesting that their particular agencies be involved as work progressed.

In the summer of 1995, Bialek and I traveled to Atlanta for a meeting with Ed Baker, Director of the Public Health Practice Office (PHPO), and Randy Gordon. Again, progress was made, and there were discussions of support for guideline development. Baker announced that the PHPO would be creating a national task force to explore the feasibility and benefit of practice guidelines for public health. We all agreed that the next step would be to select two of the four subject areas for development of the actual guidelines. Availability of an actual guideline would thus provide a model to test usefulness and applicability. These guidelines were to be created jointly by the CDC and the Public Health Guideline Development Project as advised by the Council.

Shortly before this meeting took place, the co-directors had met with a representative from the Kellogg Foundation. This foundation agreed to provide a second year of transitional funding for the project. Having an independently funded planning effort was seen as important by both the project co-directors and the foundation itself.

The project co-directors announced at the meeting in Atlanta that they intended to publish and distribute a report on the work to date. Keeping practitioners and academics apprised of the potential for practice guidelines was also seen as key to ultimate success. This report was widely circulated at the end of October 1995.

DEVELOPMENT OF GUIDELINES

As project leaders, Bialek and I regarded the agreements with the CDC and the creation of a public health service task force as major breakthroughs. Apparently the strategy of setting up an independently funded effort was having the desired effect. However, progress on the project became slower in the fall. Discussions about which two subject areas to select for development were slow to reach closure. Various CDC units in areas that coincided with those covered by the guidelines needed to be informed of the purpose of the project and required staff resources if they were to participate. Despite the evident intentions and support of both the public health service and the council for development of practice guidelines, creating an operational and collaborative work project proved difficult. Beyond the scheduling problems and technical obstacles, there were also questions about the control of guideline formation, which ultimately could have a major influence on public health practice.

I decided to set a date for a small work meeting in Baltimore to accomplish the preliminary drafting for guidelines in tuberculosis and cardiovascular disease. The leadership of these panels was invited to the meeting on December 5, 1995. Staff from the CDC were also invited.

This meeting was an informal work session concentrating on questions of the adequacy and suitability of evidence on which the guidelines were based, and on the format for presenting them. Allan Hinman, a senior CDC official, attended the meeting and apprised the group of his new responsibilities in heading guideline activities in Atlanta. Participants at the meeting were pleased by the progress and partnership that were evident. It was decided that the guideline format would consist of strategies backed by available evidence. Preliminary work in developing these evidence-based intervention strategies would be done in small work groups for both the tuberculosis and the cardiovascular areas. The broader panels were called back for a meeting in June of 1996 which resulted in draft guidelines for cardiovascular disease and tuberculosis.

EPILOGUE

The strategy of using planning study to stimulate action did facilitate movement toward the development of national guidelines. On April 1, 1996, the CDC announced the development of a guide to community preventive services. The guide is intended to complement the *Guide to Clinical Preventive Services* by focusing on community-based prevention and control strategies. The guide will be based on the best available scientific evidence and the current best thinking regarding the delineation of essential public health services and what works in the delivery of those services.

The primary target audiences of the guide will be federal, state, and local public health agencies. It is anticipated that additional users will include community-based health organizations, state Medicaid agencies, and business groups.

The CDC stated that the guide to clinical preventive services did not consider population approaches (e.g., community, occupational, and school-based approaches) to public health services. Practitioners of public health, managed care executives, health-policy makers, and payers for health care have expressed need for evidence-based recommendations, with which they can make informed decisions for selecting and implementing preventive health services within the community. The Council on Linkages between Academia and Public Health Practice, with support from the Kellogg Foundation and in collaboration with federal, state, and local public health agencies, has conducted a feasibility study entitled *Practice Guidelines for Public Health: Assessment of Scientific Evidence Feasibility and Benefits* (October, 1995). The study resulted in a consensus that "the development of public health practice guidelines would be urgently pursued." Consequently, the development of a guide to community preventive services has become a top priority.

The guide will be developed by an independent, non-federal task force on community preventive services. The task force will consist of 13 members, including the chair, appointed by the director of the CDC. Members of the task force will be drawn from multiple disciplines, including local and state health departments, managed care, behavioral science, communications sciences, epidemiology, quantitative policy analysis, decision and cost-effectiveness analysis, information systems, primary care, and management and policy. The task force will develop and apply criteria to select topics to be addressed by the guide, determine the most appropriate means of assessing evidence regarding population-based interventions, review and assess the quality of available evidence on the effectiveness and cost-effectiveness of essential community preventive health services, and develop recommendations. The complete guide is expected to be published by July 1, 2000, with individual components published as they are completed.

CHAPTER 13

Evidence of Leadership

Bobbie Berkowitz

It is very difficult if not impossible for the average man to know what he is waiting for. A warrior, however, has no problems; he knows that he is waiting for his will. [1(p.22)]

—Carlos Castañeda

The idea of becoming a warrior is an intriguing one. When a colleague introduced me to the tales of Carlos Castañeda and his teacher, Don Juan, I was struck by the power of Castañeda's perception of his ordinary and unordinary reality. The ability to perceive chance, and then to have the will to act on it and take advantage of the moment and the opportunity, is the source of my current leadership strategies. Such a process also suggests a way in which public health can create more warriors who perceive, create, and embrace opportunity. This chapter examines a case in which leadership required the ability to perceive opportunity as well as meet the challenge of balancing personal and political realities. It addresses the creation of a health reform framework in Washington State and the influence public health exerted on that process and design.

POLITICAL VERSUS PERSONAL

I believe that personal drive and the experience of success and failure are crucial to providing leadership in the policy arena. Managing the personal side of politics is a quality of leadership for which we are rarely prepared. But politics is equally important, for there are many times when one has to test policy options for their political viability. How much of our leadership do we express when we make a decision for personal reasons, telling ourselves "It's the right thing to do," rather than for political reasons? If we feel the political process will lead us to the right policy decision, what is the value of the personal side of politics and where does leadership become evident?

Promoting public health as vital to health reform requires a commitment to both public health and the principles of health reform. It requires a willingness to reform the entire system, including public health, and a vision for the "new" public health. It requires a willingness to risk current public health practice in favor of a revolution in public health. Because the change required in Washington State was monumental, we needed to believe that a collection of public health leaders could succeed in effecting such reform. My own leadership contributed to the creation and articulation of a new vision for public health. Important to my ability to lead within this environment was my willingness to cross over boundaries of current public health thinking and my decision to take certain political and personal risks, even when doing so required parting with tradition.

NEW APPOINTMENT

In the late spring of 1990, I received a call from a colleague who was involved in a grassroots organization actively engaged in health reform. He proposed that his organization submit my name to the governor to be considered for an appointment to the newly created Washington Health Care Commission. This commission would have the task of creating the framework for health reform in Washington State. I immediately accepted his offer and tapped into my network for letters and calls of support for my nomination being submitted to the governor's office. In June 1990, I took on what would become a very political role as one of 17 commissioners with the Washington Health Care Commission. (Commissioners represented health care, insurance, government, large businesses, small businesses, consumers, rural communities, legislators, human services, and labor.) At the time I was appointed, I was serving as the chief of nursing for a large metropolitan public health department. I was representing health care providers and nursing and public health staff, and I was committed to taking a broad view of health reform, including the possibility of a single-payer system.

A ROLE FOR PUBLIC HEALTH

During the first several months of my appointment, it became clear to me that my primary mission ought to be creating a role for public health within a reformed health system. At the time, the contributions the public health system could make to a healthy population were not well defined, understood, articulated, or financed. There was an opportunity for public health to participate in the work of the Washington Health Care Commission, and so I began a campaign of public health definition, awareness, articulation, and resource declaration. I wanted to make the most of this opportunity and fairly represent those who had helped me. At the same time, I needed to be focused enough to be effective. I decided that in creating a new health system, I needed to emphasize the structures, services, and systems that would lead to healthier populations. I was also very concerned about providing a voice for nurses, so that they could have influence in this new health system. If I acted effectively, nurses would be welcomed as providers and leaders within a system that recognized the value of the service itself as much as the value of who delivered it; a delivery and reimbursement system that focuses primarily on provider types rather than on services delivered may leave out crucial groups of nonphysician providers. Nurses are often excluded from decision making, not because of what they have to offer, but because of the fact that they are nurses. I took every opportunity to meet with, discuss, debate, and gain insight from groups of colleagues from nursing and public health during this process.

The process of creation and change always tempts me. This is very much the personal side of leadership. In yielding to the temptation to create, a leader needs to recognize what is achievable rather than desirable and when to ignore politics and gain important allies. In the process of creating a role for public health within health reform, I became tempted with the notion that the public health approach was the ultimate answer to the health care crisis of cost, access, and unacceptable and unaccountable quality. I had not considered the political viability of such a notion. My colleagues on the commission confirmed my vision that the approaches and values of public health were profoundly important in creating new health systems. Their reluctance in finding an "ultimate solution" was based on a lack of evidence. It is true that public health lacks a well-documented foundation for assuming leadership within the health system, and as a result, the medical care industry may discount both the system and the leaders in public health.

The Institute of Medicine report[2] on public health was quite adamant that public health was not the leader it ought to be. In spite of that, I took every opportunity to speak with my fellow commissioners and with other groups and organizations to make a case for the value and contributions of public health. I maintained that the core functions of public health were understandable and even interesting when described. Many times I worked my ideas about public health into a speech. It didn't matter who I was speaking to or what subject had been asked for; I'd find a way to mention the necessity of public health.

The need for health reform in the state of Washington was based on the premise that a growing number of residents did not have reasonable access to acute and illness care services and public health services. It troubled many that the system overemphasized the curative and did not recognize the value of addressing the actual causes of morbidity and mortality. In addition, the increase in the cost of health care had placed a substantial financial burden on individuals, families, the government, and employers. The Washington Health Care Commission believed that only fundamental reforms to the health system would address the inequities in access, cost, and quality of the health system. That the commission recognized the need for comprehensive reform and the development of a health system rather than a system of insurance reform assisted me in presenting the public health approach as an important strategy for health reform. The major barrier was the public's lack of knowledge and understanding about public health and its contribution to health improvement. The nation was focused on planning major changes in the cost and financing of health care delivery, and here in the state of Washington I was trying to get people to pay attention to prevention.

Each of my colleagues on the commission was concerned about the impact of health care costs. Each was concerned about the lack of access to and quality of health care. Ahead of the commission lay a morass: Most of the solutions to the health care crisis were complicated, many were not well documented, and some were contradictory to the goals of reform. It became tempting to limit our focus because of the number and complexity of the issues. Instead, we decided to create four committees to handle the collection, analysis, and interpretation of information and the development of recommendations. The committees addressed access, cost control, malpractice, and health services.

HEALTH SERVICES COMMITTEE

I chaired the committee on health services. This particular committee was responsible for describing the characteristics of a reformed health system and those categories of health services considered appropriate and effective in improving the population's health. We also developed recommendations for a uniform set of health services to which all residents of Washington State would have access, primarily through a uniform insurance benefits package and public health.

I specifically volunteered to chair this committee because this was where my expertise would be most valuable. It was also the committee that would influence the design of the health system. I wanted to ensure that the system would be designed to include public health as a major contributor to health improvement. I knew that if public health wasn't included in the system of services and delivery, it would not be considered in financing. I appointed two public health professionals to my committee as technical advisors, along with representatives from the medical care and human services sector of the health system.

I began meeting on a regular basis with a group of individuals interested in creating a new future for public health. This group, called the Public Health Core Functions Task Force, came together to forge a new vision for public health based on core functions and to create strategies for stable financing for the public health system. It was serendipitous that the commission work and the work of the Core Functions Task

Force were proceeding on parallel tracks. The public health community, including both state and local agencies and the university, had long been considering strategies for an improved approach to public health. The creation of the commission and my involvement in both efforts offered an opportunity to put the task force to work. We collaborated closely to develop our vision of public health, and that vision ultimately became part of the Washington Health Care Commission's recommendation to the governor of the state of Washington and to the Washington State legislature.

Conflict and Challenge

Conflict and challenge existed in three major areas. The first was in developing a consensus on the definitions of core functions of public health and articulating those definitions in ways that could communicate the purpose and value of public health. The second was in developing the financing for the public health system and gaining agreement on the appropriate level. The third was clarifying the role public health should maintain in providing clinical personal health services. I had experienced difficulties while describing the public health system to my commission colleagues. If I was unable to articulate the services public health could provide, my chance of including them in our recommendations for a uniform set of health services was limited.

The Public Health Core Functions Task Force went beyond the Institute of Medicine's report, *The Future of Public Health*,[2] and defined specifically what activities and services the core functions of public health would require. The outcome of the effort was documented in three publications: *Core Public Health Functions*,[3] *Public Health Nursing within Core Public Health Functions*,[4] and *Core Public Health Functions: Environmental Health*.[5]

Before these documents were printed, the content was transmitted to the Washington Health Care Commission through the Health Services Committee for inclusion in the final report. I know there were public health professionals who were concerned about the direction in which both the commission and the Core Functions Task Force were headed. Not everyone agreed that public health ought to be involved in health reform, nor did everyone agree that our role in public health was to embrace the core functions. We had to push ourselves constantly to consider the reality of a reformed health system that appropriately addressed the health care needs of its citizens.

Prevention, Protection, and Promotion

We knew that we could match our understanding of the role of public health with the potential reality of a reformed system by renewing our commitment to serving populations, to prevention, to health protection, and to health promotion.

At this juncture it was essential that leadership within the local public health juris-dictions and the state department of health present a unified voice. The deliberate process of the Public Health Core Functions Task Force made it possible to gain consensus; it was then my responsibility to communicate the role of public health to my colleagues on the commission. Considerable work in defining and commu-nicating the role of public health continues today in The Public Health Improve-ment Plan,[6] published by the Washington State Department of Health.

Developing an effective logic for financing the public health system required intensive effort. Our ability to put together a reasonable baseline of information on the costs of public health was hampered by lack of data. This kind of information is neither well documented nor standardized. The Washington Health Care Com-mission did recommend to the legislature that current funding for public health be doubled. The commission understood that health reform strategies designed to improve the population's health could serve as one method of reducing the overall costs of the health care system. They also understood that improving public health would require a health system that promoted the principles of prevention, protec-tion, and health promotion. When presented with data about the imbalance in funding for curative as opposed to preventive strategies, the commission took a strong stand, recommending increased funding for public health. The commission also recommended the development of the Public Health Improvement Plan (PHIP) as a way of continuing to articulate what public health financing would provide in improved public health capacity and health status improvement. The full recommendations on public health and the PHIP are contained within the Washington Health Care Commission Final Report.[7]

Whether clinical personal health services should continue to be delivered in a public health setting may have been the most difficult of all issues discussed. From my perspective on the Washington Health Care Commission, I envisioned a health system where all residents would have access to health care services through an insurance mechanism. This would free up the public health system to pursue the core functions of assessment, policy development, and assurance. I was quite sure that public health's assurance role would require our being involved in many per-sonal health services, but I did not believe that we would be heavily involved in the delivery of primary care unless the community was unable to provide a reason-able alternative. The decision to deliver clinical services from a public health set-ting would be the outcome of a community assessment process.

Most but not all public health leaders agreed with my ideas. A recommendation about who should deliver services was not articulated in the commission's report. Instead, the report detailed financing mechanisms for health care and recom-mended that clinical services be delivered through managed care and managed competition. These recommendations left the issue of clinical services within pub-lic health in need of further analysis. The opportunity to study this issue in more detail became available through publication of the report entitled Public Health Improvement Plan.[6]

LEGISLATIVE SUCCESS AND FAILURE

In November 1992, the Washington Health Care Commission's report was delivered to the governor and state legislature. When the legislative session began in January 1993, the primary health reform bill was based on the commission report. As a commissioner and the chair of the Health Services Committee, I provided legislative testimony during the next several months. I always presented the public health approach along with other detailed recommendations. When I wasn't before the legislature as a commissioner, I was there as a local public health leader, supporting the reform legislation regarding public health services. During the same time, I was appointed to my current position as deputy secretary for the Department of Health. I delayed my move to my new position until after the legislative session so I could continue to work with the legislature in a local public health capacity.

During April 1993 the final debate on health reform took place on the floor of the House of Representatives. I was overwhelmed with the desire to see a long and arduous process result in the passage of a health reform bill, and I was eager to present a new vision of public health. It was the vision of a system that made prevention a top priority, and here it was being debated in the political arena. When the vote was taken, and the bill gained final passage, I vividly remember thinking, "Now I have felt success, now I have added value." It was all very personal.

The 1993 Health Services Act that passed both the House and the Senate in Washington State was, I believe, the most comprehensive approach to health reform created at that point in the nation. Contained in that legislation was language that characterized public health by its role in core functions. Although at that time public health was still unsure of many of the specific characteristics of its future, the legislature recommended additional funding for public health, increased flexibility in funding local public health services, and a commitment to an ongoing biennial plan that would continue to articulate the standards, outcomes, finance and governance mechanisms, and resources vital to public health. These recommendations were drawn up in the Public Health Improvement Plan.[6]

Most of the 1993 Health Services Act was repealed in the 1995 legislative session. But the public health portion was retained. To see the repeal of legislation that took five years of work and dedication was a hard lesson in politics for me. Still, I was stunned that in a political environment opposed to health reform, public health emerged strengthened. I account for this phenomenon by the compelling case public health made for its role in health improvement and for the articulate message conveyed through the publication of the Public Health Improvement

Plan.[6] Nevertheless, public health services cannot improve the population's health alone. A systems approach is critical. Health reform, as envisioned by the 1990–1992 Washington State Health Care Commission, could have created such a system.

The impact of politics may result in the success or failure of the leader. I have experienced success and failure within politics using similar paths and employing many of the same strategies. I have always advised myself not to take the process and outcomes of politics personally. However, as we move through the 1990s, most issues of importance to me are debated by politicians. Undoubtedly, politics is very personal and has always been so. For myself, promoting health reform generally, and public health in particular, has become an exquisite experience resulting in personal growth. Public policy is the environment in which I struggle, achieve, and learn the most, and where I constantly question my leadership. Perhaps it is also where I have seen the strongest evidence of my leadership and warriorlike tendencies.

REFERENCES

1. Castañeda, C. *A Separate Reality: Further Conversations with Don Juan.* New York: Simon & Schuster; 1971.

2. Institute of Medicine. *The Future of Public Health*, Washington, DC: National Academy Press; 1988.

3. Washington State Core Government Public Health Functions Task Force. *Core Public Health Functions.* Olympia, WA: Washington State Dept of Health; 1993.

4. Public Health Nursing Directors of Washington, *Public Health Nursing Within Core Public Health Functions.* Olympia, WA: Washington State Dept of Health; 1993.

5. Environmental Health Directors of Washington. *Core Public Health Functions: Environmental Health.* Olympia, WA: Washington State Dept of Health; 1993.

6. Washington State Dept of Health. *The Public Health Improvement Plan.* Olympia, WA: Washington State Dept of Health; 1994.

7. Washington Health Care Commission. *Final Report.* Olympia, WA: Washington State Dept of Health; 1992.

CHAPTER 14

An Unanticipated Career in Public Health

John C. Lewin

My first awareness of the practical and critical importance of public health came to me at the beginning of my career in medicine, when I was a young physician working in northern Arizona. That moment occurred as I was watching the last outpatient of a long and demanding day leaving my clinic for home with his family. The setting included one of those breathtaking northern Arizona sunsets, its red hues spreading across the cumulus clouds atop Black Mesa, as the family pickup truck of my patient, Hosteen Todacheenie, pulled away from Kayenta Clinic. I recall feeling awed by the beauty of the environment and intrigued by the new culture in which I had been thrust. Yet I was frustrated by my realization that my medical training had insufficiently prepared me to effectively manage the health needs of my new patients.

HEALTH NEEDS AND HEALTH REALITIES

It was 1973, and I was a U.S. Public Health Service (USPHS) Commissioned Officer, a primary care physician on the Navajo Nation. Todacheenie, with his leg elevated as I had requested, rode out of sight in the back of the truck, resolutely prepared for the three-hour bouncing ride to the family hogan on a distant mesa. It was a long, uncomfortable, and expensive ride to this medical care site, the closest one available to them. I knew the chances of seeing him again in a week, as I had urgently requested, were slim.

Todacheenie had adult-onset diabetes, a common condition among the Navajo today, related both to genetic predisposition and the refined carbohydrates Navajos have increasingly consumed in modern times. I saw him that day to debride an infected ulcer on his foot. I requested that he soak the foot in hot, soapy water three times a day; and that he then air dry his foot in the sun, reapply the dressing, and keep it elevated as much as possible. I could not explain much about my dietary concerns as my spoken Navajo was limited. Unfortunately, the chances that Todacheenie would soak the foot as requested were poor, since his family had to haul their water in barrels from many miles away. Even getting him to rest and elevate his foot was unlikely, since he had to stay with his sheep as they grazed across the highlands.

I had also given Todacheenie an oral hypoglycemic medication to lower his blood sugar and an antibiotic to prevent the superficial infection from spreading. At this point in his illness, the risks of gangrene, an amputation, or a life-threatening infection were real. The modern medicines I had dispensed would easily ward off any complications, but they would be of little value in the long run. Rather than medicines, my patient needed access to modern sanitation, potable water especially; nutrition counseling and appropriate foods; and transportation to follow up health care or home care services.

I had arrived on the Navajo Nation direct from medical school and internal medicine training at the Los Angeles County-University of Southern California Medical Center. I believed that Navajos needed access to intensive and coronary care units, and that I would be able to deliver these essentials. As my memory now reconstructs those distant events, I can see the dust of the Todacheenie's truck disappearing from my mind's eye. Concurrent with that image, I remember it dawning in my awareness that an understanding of public health, my least favorite course in medical school, would yield more benefit in improving the health of the Navajo than would further investment in high-tech medical care.

GROWTH OF PUBLIC HEALTH INFRASTRUCTURE

While I continued to practice primary medical care, I became interested in working with tribal leaders and others with public health interests in the Indian Health Service to speed the development of regional wells and water and sanitation systems; to train Navajo-speaking nurses and health aides who could begin the work of public health education and nutrition programs; to establish effective disease control outreach programs for tuberculosis, venereal diseases, scarlet and rheumatic fever, and other common infectious diseases of the region; and to develop data systems and epidemiologic models to track the successes and failures of such efforts. When it was clear that the resources would not be forthcoming to bring the large numbers of physicians, nurses, and other professionals needed to extend care into the most remote areas of the reservation in New Mexico, Utah, and Arizona, we began to train community volunteers from isolated communities in the evenings in our home and in schools or chapter houses (local tribal meeting sites). This kind of training grew into the Community Health Representative

(CHR) Program, which flourishes today as a means of providing health education and community health outreach across the vast Navajo reservation and other native lands.

The public health infrastructure began to grow parallel with the health care systems, with remarkable results. Yet, with each new generation of non-Navajo physicians and administrators who arrived there from the "real world" to serve, the importance of public health had to be re-inculcated, or all the limited federal dollars would have been allocated to newer and more high-tech health care facilities and interventions.

The work on the Navajo Reservation was remarkably rich and rewarding, despite the frustrations of trying to reach so many people in dire need with such limited resources. After nearly five years as a primary physician in the Monument Valley area of northern Arizona and southern Utah, I was chosen by tribal leaders to establish and lead the Navajo Tribal Division of Health Services, the first self-determined, independent, and comprehensive Indian public health agency in America. My selection was not exactly an accident. I had been an outspoken critic of the inadequate funding and staffing of this governmental health program, based on a long-standing and only partially fulfilled treaty settlement. The Navajo leaders, no doubt, were aware of my concerns, which they clearly shared. I have always felt the responsibility to advocate for patients, either as individuals or in groups, and this sense of duty catapulted me into a new leadership role in helping the Navajo Nation.

The new Tribal Health Agency was funded by de-federalizing many millions of dollars of public health service funds to the tribe via the Indian Health Self-Determination Act. I now had the opportunity to implement that act to the fullest extent. Working on behalf of America's largest Indian tribe and living on a reservation larger than the state of West Virginia, I had become a public health leader overnight!

When I accepted this position, I recognized that the USPHS was more than a little uneasy about this transfer of money and power to the Navajo. I made it clear that I believed a Navajo public health leader needed to be recruited for long-term leadership of the agency. It took nearly two years to find the right person, but we eventually recruited an excellent leader with a master's degree in public health from the University of California at Berkeley.

In the meantime, a comprehensive public health agency had been born in the hands of an allopathic physician with no formal public health training. Fortunately, the USPHS allowed me to receive intensive training in management systems, epidemiology, and health statistics and data systems during my supposedly temporary transition from medical practice to public health administration. With these skills, some wonderful co-workers, a little luck, and a windfall of federal dollars reallocated from health care accounts to public health activities, we were able to build immunization, disease control, health promotion and education, sanitation, community health outreach, and mental health programs for nearly 200,000 Navajo people. Many of these programs are still functioning today, including the Navajo Nation's first rural bus system, built by the fledgling public health agency with federal transportation dollars, to provide patients with access to medical care from rural outposts.

SHIFT FROM MEDICAL CARE TO PUBLIC HEALTH

My wife and I had volunteered to work with the Navajo people for what we thought might be an interesting year of medical practice. Instead, we stayed nearly seven years! By the time we departed, my professional focus had necessarily shifted toward public health. I didn't recognize then that my experience in Arizona would have a profound effect on my future career, as I would become involved again and again in integrating public health and medical care in many vastly different circumstances and environments.

It was an emotionally wrenching experience for us to leave the rugged beauty and our many friends in the Navajo Nation, but we now had two small children, and we wanted to get back on track with our careers. For me, that meant going back to the private practice of medicine. We returned to our familiar home state of California and chose a community in which to settle down, but we were sidetracked by the offer of a two-week *locum tenens* (temporary substitute) medical practice in Kahului, Maui, Hawaii. Those two weeks would extend into a nearly 17-year stay in Hawaii.

I tried to ignore it, but the demanding and persistent pull of public health pursued me in this new environment. Once again I knew that I would become involved in public health policy, and once again my certainty was based on treating a particular patient whose illness seemed emblematic of a larger problem. The patient had a perplexing, undiagnosed medical condition. I recall treating an emaciated shadow of a person in his late twenties who had only recently been strikingly handsome. It was 1981, and I was a private physician in family medicine in rural Maui, as well as the medical director of a small hospital and clinic located nearly 4,000 feet above the Pacific Ocean, on the slopes of 10,000-foot Mount Haleakala.

Perhaps my memory now embellishes the scene, but I recall this patient's departure with a background of crimson clouds and the approaching sunset reflecting down on the nearby islands of Lanai and Kohoolawe. I know I watched wondering whether I could diagnose his elusive condition, which had evaded several colleagues. This young man had recently returned home to be in the care of his parents, my regular patients, after living nearly 10 years in San Francisco. Lacking health insurance, he had not received definitive or appropriate work-up or care for his strange wasting disease, associated at this point with a progressive cough and atypical chest infections. A number of medical providers in California and Hawaii had politely informed him that they couldn't continue to care for him, or order the next generation of expensive diagnostic tests he would need, without some guarantee of reimbursement. He was clearly relieved to be welcomed to our clinic.

I began to wonder if I might be seeing a case of the newly described, mysterious gay men's disease of San Francisco. Although there was no definitive test for human immunodeficiency virus (HIV) or *pneumocystis carinii* pneumonia then, this man may have been the first person in Hawaii to be diagnosed with full-blown acquired immunodeficiency syndrome (AIDS).

I took care of this patient by networking with California physicians who had already been experimenting with various therapies for *pneumocystis carinii* pneumonia and other opportunistic infections associated with HIV infection and AIDS. I finally found a research laboratory that helped me confirm the diagnosis. The patient survived several bouts of pneumonia and gastroenteritis, but finally died— relatively peacefully—at home six months later. I was with him then and throughout the course of his disease. This man and his devoted family served as a major impetus for me to become involved in Hawaii politics; my goal was to reinvigorate the languishing public health system in the state.

PUBLIC HEALTH ACTIVIST AND ADVOCATE

Public confidence in public health had fallen to a low level, in part because Hawaii's milk supplies in the late 1970s had been contaminated by heptachlor, an agricultural pesticide used in pineapple production. The department of public health had been remarkably slow to detect this problem and then appeared to attempt to cover up the evidence as it developed; moreover, it was slow to remove the contaminated milk from the market and then, under apparent pressure from the dairy industry, underestimated the risk to the public. All this is ironic because Hawaii has the oldest continuously operating public health agency in America, and before statehood Hawaii's leaders had worked very diligently for nearly a century to instill public confidence in public health. What the Hawaiian monarchs had originally regarded as a high social priority was now deemphasized by political leaders in post-statehood Hawaii for budgetary reasons.

The example of my first of many patients with AIDS raised two critical points. First, Hawaii needed a renewed commitment to public health and health education to address a threat like HIV infection and AIDS before the disease turned into a true plague. Second, even if the rest of America was not likely to act similarly, Hawaii needed to expand the access-to-health-care advantage it already had, by virtue of its "employer mandate," to achieve *universal* access, so that people like my patient could obtain the essential care they required. I became an activist and advocate in Hawaii for both causes: access to health care and public health. This occurred in part because of my experience treating Navajo people in Arizona, but also because I felt the responsibility to speak up and join hands with those public health leaders who shared my concerns, primarily the reestablishing of Hawaii's historic public health tradition and commitment.

Just as I had determined the need for action in regard to the Navajo people, I realized that important action was needed in Hawaii. I began to share my feelings with physician colleagues, community leaders, and elected officials long before anything dramatic actually happened. Because I had practiced medicine in Kayenta, Arizona, one of the most remote places in the contiguous states, for nearly five years before Navajo leaders asked me to develop and lead their first public health agency, I knew that it takes time to convince people of the need for a major change in direction. In fact, political leaders typically will not support major change unless their constituents are demanding it. One needs to be persistent, insistent, and willing to risk offending the status quo.

In Hawaii, change did not come quickly either. As a primary care doctor in a rural part of Maui, far from Hawaii's political center in Honolulu, I advocated a health care and public health renaissance in Hawaii for nearly seven years before anybody other than a few close colleagues noticed. Nonetheless, my wife Sandra and I founded the Wellth Institute in Maui in 1982, through which we organized numerous public forums on topics related to community health issues, environmental responsibility, and the future of medicine. Speakers, first mainly from Hawaii, then from around the nation and the world, came to Maui to hypothesize about the future of health and society. It was a stimulating and entertaining side activity, but as a very busy primary care physician, I didn't have much time to convert ideas into social and political action.

Several years later, the chance for action came. In late 1986, Hawaii elected its first governor of Hawaiian ancestry, John D. Waiheé III. Governor Waiheé apparently agreed with my vision of Hawaii as the "Health State" and subscribed to my plea for a resurgence of public health leadership. He asked me to move to Honolulu and become the State Director of Health. I balked at first, finding it very difficult to leave my practice and the wonderful life we had created for ourselves on Maui, which now included three children.

After long consideration of many factors, including the reality that public health leaders do not earn an income comparable to that of most practicing physicians, I accepted the position of Hawaii's Director of Health. We moved to Honolulu in January 1987. In this cabinet-level role, I directed all public health activities, served as chief executive officer for one of the nation's largest public hospital systems, administered mental health and substance abuse programs, and managed the state's environmental protection activities. The time was right. Governor Waiheé was supportive, the public was ready, and there was a true renaissance of public health during the nearly eight-year period during which I had the privilege of leading the Hawaii's multitalented health department.

During this time I also became nationally involved in public health as president of the Association of State and Territorial Health Officials and as a board member of the Partnership for Prevention and of the Public Health Foundation of Washington, D.C. When Hawaii suddenly received media and policy attention because of its expanded health access, I became very involved with Congress and the Clinton administration regarding increased coverage of the uninsured and the opportunity for integration of health care and public health in the reform process. Clinton's health plan was largely based on the Hawaiian health system.

HAWAII'S HEALTH SYSTEM

In Hawaii, we were able to expand coverage from employer's mandated base levels to include clinical preventive services, mental health services, and substance abuse services. We developed the State Health Insurance Program to provide affordable and guaranteed private coverage to the remaining uninsured populations in Hawaii. We developed models for extending seamless benefits coverage by linking Medicaid, workers' compensation coverage, and private insurance. These accomplishments enabled us to participate in various key roles in the national health system reform discussions.

Throughout the health reform debates of 1993 and 1994, Hawaii was able to recognize the importance of maintaining and building the public health infrastructure and safety net as an essential part of improving and protecting America's health status. Hawaii developed the nation's first statewide anonymous testing systems, mandatory statewide school educational programs, state-subsidized early treatment programs, and strict confidentiality-protection laws dealing with HIV infection and AIDS. Hawaii developed highly aggressive and successful programs dealing with hepatitis B and other sexually transmitted diseases. The result has been significant reductions of new infections and reduced morbidity and mortality from these and other infectious diseases.

Hawaii's department of health has also implemented the nation's most successful approaches to preventing child abuse and neglect and has been aggressive in the early detection and intervention of childhood disabilities. Hawaii has some of the nation's strongest anti-tobacco legislation and one of the highest tobacco taxes. Public health accomplishments have often gone hand-in-hand with health access interventions.

PERSONAL CHANGES

While I had never had the time to pursue a public health degree, my various roles as a practicing physician, public health leader, hospital system administrator, environmental leader, and health policy specialist have emphasized the importance of public health in my career. As an associate professor of international health at the University of Hawaii, I was given the opportunity to share my experience and ideas with public health students. Students need to understand that public health has reluctantly become a major voice, only asserting the provision of primary medical care to the indigent, the frail, and the uninsured in the past two decades. The irony is that public health may now resist the opportunity of phasing out its emphasis on health care delivery as reform toward providing universal access progresses, so as to be able to refocus on the neglected public health needs of America. If public health is going to finance its core public health responsibilities, it now needs to find a way to partner with medical care, where all the health-related money is being spent. Public health needs health care funding and must apply its skills in prevention, biostatistics, and epidemiology to improve health care's return on investment.

Meanwhile, the emergence of capitated managed care is pushing physicians, hospitals, and health care systems into awareness of population-based community health care, a foreign domain that they have had little desire to explore until now. The irony of these parallel developments is that a marriage between public health and Western medicine is, in my view, a social, financial, and professional imperative.

By the end of my eight-year tenure as Hawaii's Director of Health, I was the longest-surviving top state-level health official in all 50 states. This is a commentary on the politically demanding nature of public health service. I had become a well-known public person in Hawaii by virtue of the extensive media coverage I had received while managing the health and environmental affairs of the state. In the spring of 1994, a group of respected friends and business and community leaders tried to convince me to take a bold step; now that the incumbent governor had reached his two-term legal limit in office, they thought I should run for the office of governor myself. Skeptical at first about my chances of success, and concerned about the effects of such a venture on my family, I finally threw my hat in the ring for what would become a closely contested race. To come so close to winning in my first run for public office, despite being a late entry, was a remarkably rewarding experience for myself and the entire family.

After the election, I started a health policy consulting firm and considered resuming my clinical practice as a part-time avocation. My consulting activities became increasingly demanding, both in California, where for-profit managed care was wreaking havoc on physicians, hospitals, and patients, and also in the Asia and Pacific region, where both health care and public health activities were greatly expanding. In the course of these activities, I agreed to be interviewed for the position of chief executive officer for the California Medical Association, headquartered in San Francisco. While at first I saw this as a consulting opportunity, I became aware that the solutions to the challenges that had been my lifelong concerns, namely providing universal access to health care and furthering public health, would likely receive attention in the volatile and dynamic California environment. I accepted the position.

I now often find myself commuting to San Francisco from Marin County by ferryboat. I am the chief executive officer and executive vice-president of the California Medical Association (CMA) with its 38,000 physicians and seven subsidiary corporations. On the surface, it seems that this chapter in my life is devoted exclusively to health care, where organized medicine has traditionally focused its attention. And, in fact, in the past six months we have launched a new statewide health plan, California Advantage, that intends to transform profits into improved quality of care and healthier communities. The plan was created specifically for physicians to compete fairly and effectively in the marketplace. We also hope to counter the adverse effects on patient care, including the rising numbers of uninsured persons, associated with the emerging business model of profit-driven health plans in California. We have created a new foundation to study health outcomes and to determine the means of more effectively monitoring changes in the health status of populations. We have created the Institute for Medical Quality to evaluate and accredit health plans and medical facilities on the basis of cost *and* quality. There may be a touch of interest in public health care in each of these projects, but they are mainly focused on health care systems.

Currently, much energy has been expended by the rapidly changing CMA in preventing the public health safety net in Los Angeles and other counties from collapsing. The CMA is exploring new models that would use MediCal (California's Medicaid) resources more efficiently to be able to expand coverage to nearly seven million uninsured persons. We are using considerable legislative and legal muscle to prevent repeal of mandatory motorcycle helmet laws, to expand nonsmokers' rights in the workplace, and to further raise the tobacco tax.

FUTURE PATHS?

I can't foresee where this very challenging and exciting aspect of my career will lead. I suspect it may help me develop the skills needed to bring about the marriage of public health and medicine. It has to, because the survival and successful evolution of both disciplines depends on this awkward union. Everybody in health care and in public health is going to have to accept major change in the next few years, even though in both camps heels are dug in. I would love to push both disciplines toward a common goal. Perhaps that is what my career has been all about: attempting to motivate colleagues to climb the ladder just as far as they are willing and able. It may be time to ask them to climb just a few more rungs. And why not? There is reason to be optimistic. In 1996 the nation is spending more than $4000 per man, woman, and child each year for health care. If we can solve such problems as administrative waste, inappropriate and ineffective care, the failure to apply the principles of prevention, and the corporate profiteerism that characterizes health care today, resources are sufficient to accommodate universal access to health care and to construct a public health safety net.

I am pondering a strange meeting I recently held in my new office overlooking the San Francisco Bay. It was attended by leaders of medicine, academia, and various associations dedicated to fighting tobacco use and preventing tobacco-related disease. The group was angry and frustrated at the failure to reach a consensus.

There has been a three-year dispute in California about how to allocate the diminishing tax resources resulting from Proposition 99 (Prop 99), the 1987 initiative that added 25 cents to the price of a pack of cigarettes. The revenues are divided up according to a formula that applies the monies to indigent health care, anti-tobacco education, tobacco-related disease research, and an environmental project. During recent years, California has been experiencing a severe budgetary deficit and has had to cut back on indigent health care and public health services. At the same time, the Prop 99 revenues were diminishing because fewer people were smoking. Then a crisis occurred over how to prioritize the Prop 99 funds. Hospitals, a majority of physicians, children's advocates, and safety net health providers favored maintaining indigent health care funding for children and young mothers at the previous funding levels and taking the necessary reductions out of anti-tobacco education and research programs until the state budget improved. A long and increasingly nasty political battle ensued, and parties that should be aligned are now bitter enemies because they cannot agree on which constituencies and which organizations will incur the cuts in funding. The fight over diminishing Prop 99 resources has precluded forming a strategic alliance that would raise taxes to a more appropriate level or would seek general funds to relieve the stress on the programs funded by the diminishing tobacco tax revenues. Meanwhile, our common enemy, the tobacco industry, must be laughing loudly.

Unlike some of the organizations involved in this debacle, physicians in the CMA find themselves in a profound dilemma: whether to support public health education against tobacco use or to support access to essential care for indigent persons. Doctors consider both goals noble, even critical, to health care, although the immediate concerns of poor women and children seem more pressing.

I am beginning to understand better what my role must be. I am experiencing again the perennial competition for scarce resources, that tension between the need to provide universal access to health care and the need to rebuild and strengthen the public health safety net. My career has been representative of both the problem and the solution. We are always asked to choose between health care for the indigent and public health needs, and we are told that only one or the other can be emphasized. But my career has made it clear to me that this view is absolutely and fundamentally wrong, financially disastrous, and ethically unacceptable. Instead, we must choose public health *and* access to essential health care. We must find a way to do *both*.

Index